The Radically Honest Guide to Fertility Treatment

Navigate the process and take back control

Dr Louise Goddard-Crawley
& Jules McDonald

GREEN TREE
LONDON • OXFORD • NEW YORK • NEW DELHI • SYDNEY

GREEN TREE
Bloomsbury Publishing Plc
50 Bedford Square, London, WC1B 3DP, UK
Bloomsbury Publishing Ireland Limited,
29 Earlsfort Terrace, Dublin 2, D02 AY28, Ireland

First published in Great Britain 2026

A catalogue record for this book is available from the British Library

Library of Congress Cataloguing-in-Publication data has been applied for

ISBN: TPB: 978-1-3994-2829-3; ePUB: 978-1-3994-2827-9; ePDF: 978-1-3994-2828-6

2 4 6 8 10 9 7 5 3 1

Typeset in IBM Plex Serif by Lumina Datamatics Ltd
Printed and bound in Great Britain by Clays Ltd, Elcograf S.p.A.

To find out more about our authors and books visit www.bloomsbury.com
and sign up for our newsletters
For product safety related questions contact productsafety@bloomsbury.com

For Nicky and Andrew. Thank you for your creativity, your wisdom and your endless support. You believed in this book and in us, and you stood beside us every step of the way. Your encouragement carried us through the long nights, the difficult chapters and the emotional weight of writing a book that means so much to so many. We are grateful beyond words.

We have written this book . . .

For our children Archie and Mara – you are the reason our hearts remain soft, hopeful and full. This book is for you, and for every family built through courage, perseverance, medicine and love. Born through the hope of assisted reproduction, you are a reminder of what is possible when science and love come together.

For all those who are going through, have gone through or are about to embark on the journey of fertility treatment – you are brave, and this path is undeniably difficult.

For all those who have faced loss – we honour your courage and send our deepest compassion for all you have endured.

Contents

About the authors

Dr Louise Goddard-Crawley is a consultant psychologist and former fertility nurse whose career has been dedicated to supporting individuals and couples through the emotional, relational and physical realities of fertility treatment. She specialises in the psychological side of fertility and health, drawing on many years of clinical experience to help people feel understood, steadied and informed during what can be one of the most vulnerable periods of their lives. Louise's doctoral research explored the emotional and psychological complexities of unexplained infertility, and her work now centres on clear communication, compassionate guidance and helping people make sense of complex medical information in a way that feels human and manageable.

Jules McDonald has spent more than 22 years nursing and 17 years working in reproductive medicine and has led patient care and operational services across respected IVF centres in the United Kingdom and UAE, helping shape the future of fertility care, patient experience and reproductive health standards. Having also experienced parts of the fertility journey personally and within her own family, Jules brings a rare combination of professional expertise and genuine empathy to her work. Known for her calm presence, warmth and patient-centred approach, she has supported thousands of individuals and couples through some of the most emotional and life-changing moments of their lives. Her leadership is grounded not only in clinical excellence and operational experience, but in a deep commitment to ensuring every patient feels heard, respected and cared for.

Introduction
Our message to you

Before we begin, we want to meet you exactly where you are. Whether you are hopeful, uncertain, overwhelmed or simply searching for clarity, you deserve a space where things are explained honestly, kindly and without assumptions. One guiding belief shaped this book from the very start: if information is power, then education is key – and for too long, people seeking fertility support have been denied it. You should not have to navigate this journey in the dark. You deserve to understand your body, your options and what all the jargon around fertility, treatment and pregnancy actually means.

And that is what we are here to help with.

In the past, doctors were seen as experts who should not be questioned. Patients, especially women, were expected to be passive and agreeable, to accept that the doctor knew best and to follow treatment plans without being given a clear explanation.

Take the pill, for example. Many of us were prescribed it for painful periods without ever being told we were essentially inducing a chemical menopause. What are the long-term effects of this? How does starting and stopping the pill shape our bodies over time? These are important questions that have been overlooked and under-researched. Yet we were expected to take the treatment without asking why.

In some ways, things have changed. We are more informed and less willing to allow our bodies to be managed without explanation. But in many ways, we are still in the dark – especially when it comes to fertility.

Fertility issues are more common than many people realise, impacting approximately one in six people. These challenges can arise from various factors that can affect anyone, regardless of sex or gender. Common causes include hormonal imbalances, structural issues of the reproductive organs and problems with sperm or egg quality.

However, here in the United Kingdom, fertility treatment is surrounded by barriers. The NHS offers treatment in limited circumstances; even then, eligibility depends on where you live, local funding and strict criteria. Many people are forced to turn to private clinics at significant personal cost. The private fertility industry continues to grow, yet patients often tell us they feel misinformed, financially pressured and unclear about their real chances of success.

In our clinical careers, we have seen all of this first-hand. We have spent decades working in reproductive health. We have seen people arrive anxious, hopeful, confused and underprepared, and we have seen how a lack of clear information can turn a challenging journey into a frightening one. Much of the distress people feel is caused not by their bodies but by the silence, mixed messages and missing information around them.

The uncertainty so many people feel is not abstract. It appears at the exact moments that matter most. Deciding whether to start treatment. Choosing a clinic and a team you can trust. Weighing protocols, tests and add-ons. Making sense of success rates. Considering genetics. Exploring donor options. Working out how to fund everything. Deciding when to continue and when to stop. Without clear, plain-spoken guidance, these decisions can feel impossible. How could they not?

Traditional narratives paint the journey to parenthood as a fairy tale. But the reality for many people is far more complicated. There is loss here: not only the loss of pregnancy, but also the loss of things working the way you imagined they would.

For too long, fertility medicine has been wrapped in comforting stories that do not always match reality. You may have been told that treatment is straightforward or that success is simply a matter of time. When the reality turns out to be harder than expected, you are left wondering why no one prepared you. Fertility treatment can be emotionally, physically and financially demanding. That is not because you have failed. It is because the system has not supported you well enough.

We believe this needs to change. And there are two parts to that change.

The first is better research and better testing so reproductive medicine can understand the body in all its complexity. That kind of progress requires time, policy, investment and international effort.

The second part, the one that can change right now, is communication. The way in which information is shared. The clarity and honesty people are offered. The support they receive at each stage. This is the part of the system we can influence. And that is why we have written *The Radically Honest Guide to Fertility Treatment*.

What this book offers

In our day-to-day work, much of what we do is help people understand what is happening to them on their fertility journey. We spend time relieving confusion, easing fear and repairing the harm caused by rushed or unclear explanations. We see the same themes every week: overwhelm, gaps in understanding and people being asked to cope without having the full picture.

This book is our way of placing that missing clarity into your hands. It brings together everything we have learned from thousands of one-to-one conversations. It offers the honesty, steadiness and guidance you should have received from the beginning. Throughout our careers, we have heard the same sentences again and again:

- 'If only I'd known.'
- 'I wish someone had told me.'
- 'Why does no one talk about this?'

These words usually appear after the hardest experiences. Fertility struggles. Failed treatment cycles. Pregnancy loss. Months of uncertainty. Confusion created by vague or inconsistent information. You might have had some of these thoughts yourself:

- *If only I knew how success rates were calculated.*
- *If only I knew that age affects egg* quality *more than egg* quantity.
- *If only I knew that endometriosis and polyendocrine metabolic ovarian syndrome (PMOS) can affect fertility and they need proper investigation.*
- *If only I knew how much time, money and emotional energy treatment demands.*
- *If only I knew how the medication would make me feel.*
- *If only I knew that using a donor or choosing to stop treatment is not failure but a form of courage.*

We have written this book to help turn those words into something different. Not *If only I knew!* but *Now I understand, and I know what to do next!*

You deserve clarity, honesty and compassionate information that supports you to make confident decisions about your body, your treatment and your future.

Drawing on our combined experience in reproductive health, we have created a guide that helps you navigate the medical aspects, practical demands and emotional reality of fertility treatment. Our intention is not to frighten you or offer false reassurance. Our intention is to tell you the truth kindly and help you feel prepared, informed and supported.

In this book, you will find a clear understanding of your body, your fertility and the treatment options available to you. We take you both through everything step by step, from how your menstrual cycle works to what the different tests and treatments involve for both of you and the decisions you may face along the way. We explain the medical information in simple language, help you make sense of the emotional impact and offer steady guidance, so you feel supported rather than overwhelmed. Our hope is that by the time you finish, you feel informed, grounded and more in control of a process that often leaves people confused and unsure of where to turn. Knowledge will not remove every difficulty, but it can make the path clearer and kinder. That is what we want for you: to feel as though you are taking back some control.

Before we begin, we want you both to know something important about how we approach this topic. We are guided by trusted organisations such as the World Health Organization (WHO), the Human Fertilisation & Embryology Authority (HFEA) and the European Society of Human Reproduction and Embryology (ESHRE), but also – and just as importantly – by our own lived experience and decades of work with thousands of patients across fertility clinics. We have seen every shape this journey can take, every question, every frustration and every moment of quiet hope. Our aim is to give you not simply evidence-based information but also the kind of understanding that only comes from years of walking this path with others.

If knowledge is power, then education is one of the kindest forms of support you can offer yourself; we believe that with all our hearts.

This guide can be read as a whole, or you can scan some sections while paying more attention to others that feel more relevant to you. As with all things fertility, a one-size-fits-all approach does not work.

Sending our love and support,

Jules and Louise x

A note about language and triggers

As medical professionals, we carefully consider the words we use. The term 'infertility' can be off-putting, as it implies the *presence* of something (like a disease) rather than the *absence* of something (like a baby). It can also sound like a permanent state, when for many it is temporary. For some people, 'childless not by choice' or 'involuntarily without children' might seem more fitting.

We are still exploring this terminology. We may never find a definitive answer to what phrase is most appropriate, as what resonates for one person might not work for another. To us, 'fertility challenges' sounds gentler than 'infertility'. Throughout this book, we aim to avoid language that triggers negative emotions or makes what you are experiencing sound like a disease. If we make mistakes, please forgive us. Our intention is always, as Hippocrates wisely said, to do no harm.

In many settings, especially medical ones, you will often hear the word miscarriage. Many people find that word difficult because it can sound as though something has gone wrong with the way the pregnancy was carried. Although that is not what the term is intended to mean medically, it can land as though the body has somehow failed. Increasingly, clinicians and support organisations are using the term pregnancy loss instead. This places the emphasis on the experience of loss rather than on the idea that something has gone wrong.

In this book we will use the term pregnancy loss where possible because it better reflects the reality we see every day in fertility care. Most of the time these events are not the result of something a person did or did not do. They are the result of biological processes that sit far outside anyone's control. Using the language of loss acknowledges both the grief that can accompany these experiences and the fact that they are rarely the consequence of personal failure.

If you feel triggered by any of the information in this guide, take a minute. Be gentle and be kind to yourself, and seek support from loved ones or a professional. Reach out to a partner or friend, or find a fertility buddy – someone who is also going through this journey. If necessary, put the book down and take some time for self-care. It's okay to ask for help and prioritise your wellbeing. Remember to take care of yourself and know that we are here to support you through this journey.

Furthermore, fertility treatments and medical interventions for fertility struggles are often grouped under the term 'in vitro fertilisation' (IVF), but IVF itself is just one of many available treatments. In this book, we will discuss all of these options with you, from the broader concept of IVF to more specific and nuanced treatments. Each approach brings its own challenges and possibilities; by exploring them together, we hope to demystify the process and provide a clearer understanding of the paths available.

Inclusivity statement

As we present this guide to fertility treatment, we want to acknowledge that the language and examples may at times feel centred around heterosexual couples. This is not a reflection of our beliefs but rather an attempt to offer a clear overview of treatment options and processes. We understand that fertility journeys are experienced by a diverse range of individuals and couples, including LGBTQ+ families, single parents by choice and others whose paths may differ from traditional narratives. The nuances of inclusivity in fertility care are crucial. This book is intended as a broad resource, and we fully recognise the need for more specific guidance for all groups seeking fertility treatment.

1

Understanding your body: your eggs, your hormones and the cycle that makes pregnancy possible

So much of fertility medicine can feel technical and overwhelming, and it is very hard to make sense of anything later on unless you first understand what your body is quietly trying to do each month. This chapter is about giving you that foundation in a way that feels clear, respectful and genuinely helpful. Let's begin.

Why we are explaining this

Before we explore why pregnancy might not be happening for you, we want to help you truly understand what should ideally be happening and what your body is designed to do. So many women come to us feeling confused, frightened or ashamed, and almost all of them say the same thing: 'I never really learned how my menstrual cycle works.'

We absolutely do not want this to sound patronising. The truth is, most women reach adulthood without being taught the basics. Even we, as women, as nurses and now as authors, did not properly understand our own hormones or menstrual cycles until we began working in fertility. That is how poorly reproductive health is taught across the world. We had to learn this, and we want to help you understand it too.

If you do not know this information, you are not behind, you are not silly and it is not your fault. Learning it now is a gift you are giving yourself. We are walking beside you, woman to woman, nurse to patient, sharing the knowledge we wish someone had given us years ago.

Let's go through this together.

Understanding your period and your menstrual cycle

Having a period is one of the few experiences almost everyone with ovaries shares, even though most of us have never been taught what it truly means. For many, it becomes something to tolerate, hide or simply get through. But your period is your body's monthly reset. It marks the start of a new menstrual cycle and gives you a reliable point from which everything else flows.

DEFINITIONS

A **menstrual cycle** begins with the first day of a period and ends the day before the next one starts. Each cycle typically lasts around 28 days, though anything between about 21 and 35 days is considered common.

A **period** is just one part of the menstrual cycle: the bleeding phase, when the lining of the uterus (or womb) is shed because pregnancy has not occurred (*see* below for more details).

Ovulation is when one ovary releases an egg. This usually happens once during each menstrual cycle. After the egg is released, it travels down the fallopian tube, where it can meet sperm and be fertilised. If the egg is not fertilised, the body prepares for a period.

Many people use the terms 'period' and 'menstrual cycle' interchangeably. In this book, when we talk about a 'menstrual cycle' or a 'cycle', we mean the whole process your body goes through each month; when we refer to a period, we specifically mean the bleeding phase.

What a period actually is

A period is your body letting go of the uterine lining it has built during your menstrual cycle. Throughout each menstrual cycle, your hormones prepare the lining to welcome a possible pregnancy. If pregnancy does not happen, your hormone levels fall. That drop tells your uterus, very gently and naturally, 'We don't need this lining this month.' The lining then breaks down and leaves your body as menstrual blood, also known as your period.

Just like the people who have them, periods come in all shapes and sizes. Some are light, some are heavy; some arrive like clockwork, others prefer to wander. Some last a couple of days, others stretch out. There is no single right version. Your period is simply your body's own normal, and understanding that normal is far more useful than comparing yourself to anyone else.

A period is not your body failing. It is your body completing a menstrual cycle. It means you have ovulated or attempted to ovulate, your hormones have communicated and your cycle is beginning again. In the simplest terms, during each menstrual cycle:

- Your body prepares.
- Your body checks whether pregnancy has happened.
- If it hasn't, it resets.
- That reset is your period. Your cycle is complete.
- Your body prepares again . . .

And while your period can be frustrating, painful or inconvenient, it is also a sign that your body is working in rhythm. This is why we suggest tracking your menstrual cycle (*see* below). When you understand your own rhythm rather than guessing or stressing, everything becomes a little clearer and a lot kinder.

HOW TO TRACK YOUR MENSTRUAL CYCLE

Start by noting the first day of each period. This is the most important reference point, as it marks day one of your menstrual cycle. You should also note when your period ends, which helps you understand your period's length. Over a few months, the natural pattern of your cycle will emerge.

You do not need apps or charts unless they genuinely help you. A few gentle notes are enough to give you a clearer sense of your menstrual cycle.

Later in this chapter, we will explore other aspects of your cycle that you can consider tracking to understand when your fertile window is likely to fall (*see* pp. 22–24).

All of this is helping you tune in to your body and the quiet shifts it moves through, so you can see just how much work it does for you every single menstrual cycle. You cannot stop these shifts, but you can learn to recognise them and work with them. As stress-reduction expert Jon Kabat Zinn says, 'You can't stop the waves, but you can learn to surf.'

As you begin to recognise the rhythm of your menstrual cycle, you are also starting to understand what your ovaries are quietly working on month after month. This brings us to the part many of us were never taught about: your eggs.

The story of your eggs

Your relationship with your eggs began long before you were born. When you were still developing inside your mother's uterus, your ovaries held around 6,000,000–7,000,000 immature eggs. By birth, that number had already fallen to 1,000,000–2,000,000. By puberty, when your periods began, you had around 300,000–500,000 eggs remaining.

And it goes back even further than that. When your grandmother was pregnant with your mother, the tiny cells that would one day become you were already forming inside your mother's ovaries; this means you, your mother and your grandmother all shared the same biological environment for a moment in time.

As the years pass, the number of eggs gradually continues to fall. At around 35 years of age, the average woman has roughly 25,000 eggs left. By the time menopause arrives, usually around the age of 50 or 51, only around 1,000 remain.

This natural decline in the number of eggs you have is not something you caused by stressing, working, waiting or living imperfectly. Your ovaries have been quietly using eggs every single month since before you took your first breath. In most menstrual cycles, only one egg is released. Other eggs that briefly begin to develop are naturally reabsorbed by the body. Although this chapter focuses on eggs and ovarian biology, fertility is never solely a woman's journey. Partners often experience the uncertainty, hope, grief and decision-making alongside them, and male fertility factors contribute to around half of all fertility challenges. Fertility treatment works best when both people feel informed, included and supported throughout the process.

> **Radical honesty: You do not need thousands of eggs to become pregnant. You need one good egg each menstrual cycle, as well as a body whose hormones are communicating properly.**

Next, let's have a look at what happens hormonally during a typical menstrual cycle.

The hormonal dance

Your menstrual cycle is a beautifully orchestrated conversation between your brain and your ovaries. This conversation repeats itself every cycle and moves through three phases: the follicular phase, ovulation and the luteal phase.

The follicular phase (period to ovulation)

The first day of your period marks the beginning of your menstrual cycle. As the lining that had built during the previous cycle sheds, your brain releases a hormone called follicle-stimulating hormone (FSH). FSH gently wakes up your ovaries and encourages your eggs to start growing.

One egg begins to take the lead. As it develops, it produces the hormone oestrogen. Oestrogen thickens the lining of your uterus, creating a warm, cushioned environment for a possible embryo (a fertilised egg, created when an egg and sperm fuse). It also changes your cervical mucus, making it more fluid so sperm can travel more easily. This entire phase is about preparation, and it varies in length for every woman.

Ovulation (the moment of possibility)

Once the leading egg is mature, your brain releases a powerful surge of luteinising hormone (LH), which tells the ovary to release the egg. This moment is ovulation, when the egg leaves the ovary and begins its journey into the fallopian tube.

Ovulation itself is brief. The egg usually survives for around 12–24 hours after being released. Sperm, however, can live inside the body for up to five days. This is why pregnancy is possible across a small window of time (known as the 'fertile window') rather than on one exact day. This fertile window spans roughly six days. It includes the five days leading up to ovulation and the day on which ovulation occurs. If sperm are already present when the egg is released, fertilisation can happen.

> **Radical honesty: Here is the part that people are never told: the fertile window includes the five days before ovulation and the day of ovulation itself, and most pregnancies happen because of intercourse before ovulation happens, not on ovulation day.**

Because ovulation timing can shift from cycle to cycle, focusing on a single calendar day is often misleading. You may have heard that day 14 is the 'best' or 'magic' day to conceive. This idea comes from a 'textbook' 28-day menstrual cycle, where ovulation happens roughly halfway through. In reality, this is an average, not a rule. This is why understanding your own cycle matters. We explain this in more detail later in this chapter (*see* pp. 19–20).

Your body may give you a natural sign that ovulation is approaching through changes in your cervical mucus. Around this time, cervical mucus often becomes clear, slippery and stretchy, similar to raw egg whites. If you touch it, it may stretch into a long, stringy thread. Some women notice this every month, some only occasionally and some not at all. All of these patterns are normal.

The luteal phase (after ovulation)

After the egg is released, the ovary produces the hormone progesterone. Progesterone stabilises and nourishes the uterine lining, making it soft and receptive if an embryo arrives. You may feel warmer, more tired or slightly different emotionally during this phase. That is progesterone doing its job.

If pregnancy occurs, progesterone levels stay high. If pregnancy does not occur, progesterone gently falls, and that drop triggers your next period. This phase is usually around 12–14 days long. And this is where your experience often shifts from physical to emotional.

How your body and mood move together each menstrual cycle

You might notice your mood shifting across your menstrual cycle, often in ways that feel sudden or confusing. In the first half of your cycle (the follicular phase, leading up to ovulation), rising oestrogen levels can make you feel clearer, more focused or just a little more like yourself. You may feel more social, more motivated or more open to connection. This is your biology supporting you, not a coincidence.

In the second half, when progesterone takes the lead in the luteal phase, things often feel different. You may feel softer, slower or more easily overwhelmed. You might find that your tolerance is lower, your emotions sit closer to the surface or you need more rest than usual. This is not you being dramatic or too sensitive. This is your body doing exactly what it is designed to do as it prepares for the possibility of pregnancy.

And when progesterone levels drop at the end of the cycle, it can bring a wave of sudden emotion or irritability: a sense that everything feels harder or heavier. Many women describe this as feeling unlike themselves, but really it is just the hormonal tide going out.

None of this means you are unstable or overreacting. It means you are human. It means your body is responding to its hormonal rhythm, a rhythm that has been unfolding inside you long before you even knew what a menstrual cycle was.

When you understand what is happening, it becomes easier to meet yourself with patience rather than criticism. Instead of wondering, *What's wrong with me?* you can recognise that your body is moving through its natural monthly rhythm. And when you can name what is happening, you can respond to yourself more gently, with steadiness rather than frustration.

The cycle that makes pregnancy possible

We want you to understand how your body works before we talk about why pregnancy might not be happening, because without this foundation, it is impossible to make sense of what might be going wrong. You cannot make sense of potential problems unless you first understand the system itself: your eggs, your hormones, your fertile window and the rhythm your body moves through each menstrual cycle.

When we say 'the cycle that makes pregnancy possible', we are talking about your menstrual cycle, which is a very specific and delicate sequence of events. Pregnancy can only happen when several things align at the right moment:

- An egg is selected, grows (matures) and is released.
- Your hormones rise and fall in a coordinated pattern.
- Your uterine lining grows in a healthy, receptive way.
- The sperm meet the egg within hours of ovulation.
- The embryo reaches the uterus at the right stage.
- The lining is ready to accept it.

It is easy to forget that every menstrual cycle, your body quietly tries to make this happen without you needing to do anything at all. The process is not random. It is a biological story with a beginning, a middle and an end.

A cycle that makes pregnancy possible is one in which all of the steps happen in order, with timing that allows the egg, sperm and uterine lining to meet each other at the right moment. It is not about being perfect. It is not about doing everything right. It is about your hormones communicating well, your ovary releasing an egg and your uterine lining responding as it should.

It is important to remember that a 'normal' menstrual cycle is not always the generally accepted 28-day cycle. Cycles differ from woman to woman. A cycle that makes pregnancy possible can be 24 days long, 33 days long or anything in between. What matters is that the cycle includes all of the following:

- An egg being matured.
- Ovulation actually happening.
- Sufficient oestrogen to prepare the lining.
- Sufficient progesterone to support the fertilised egg.

When even one part of this sequence is disrupted, pregnancy becomes less likely. Not impossible, but simply less likely. This is where understanding is powerful. Without knowledge, it is easy to assume your body is failing you. With knowledge, you can see that the system is complex, finely tuned and often doing far more right than wrong.

CASE STUDY: AMELIA AND GEORGE – THE COUPLE WHO THOUGHT SOMETHING WAS WRONG WITH THEM

Amelia and George had been trying to conceive for several months when they began to worry that something was wrong. Amelia's menstrual cycles were irregular (sometimes 26 days, sometimes 35), and she convinced herself this meant her body was not working properly. George tried to reassure her, but both of them carried a quiet fear that they were facing something serious.

They avoided talking to friends because everyone else seemed to have predictable menstrual cycles and clear patterns. Each month, they tried around day 14 because that was what they had heard was 'normal'. When nothing happened, Amelia blamed her body and George blamed himself, even though neither of them said it out loud.

It wasn't until Amelia began noting the first day of each period that a pattern emerged. Her cycles weren't random at all, just longer than the textbook 28 days. She started paying attention to her cervical mucus and realised she consistently showed signs of ovulation around day 21, not day 14.

For the first time, Amelia felt in sync with her body rather than ashamed of it. She began to understand that irregular does not mean broken, and that her cycle was simply operating on its own timetable. George said it felt like the fog had lifted, and they finally had something to trust instead of guessing.

They didn't conceive immediately, but their whole experience changed. Amelia no longer felt betrayed by her body, and George no longer felt helpless. They felt like partners again, learning something new together rather than blaming themselves in silence.

This shift didn't remove every challenge, but it turned fear into understanding and doubt into clarity. Sometimes, the most powerful change comes from learning how your body actually works rather than how you think it should work.

How to try to conceive naturally

Before we begin, we want to gently acknowledge that if you are reading this book, there is a good chance you are already past this stage. You might be months or years into trying. You might already be exploring investigations or treatment. You might already feel exhausted by the idea of 'just trying naturally', especially if that advice has ever been given to you casually or without care.

We see you. We respect where you are. And we are not asking you to go backwards.

The reason this chapter is here is that we want this book to support every person at every point in their journey. Some are just beginning. Some are trying naturally between treatments. Some are starting again after loss. And some simply want to understand their body better for the first time.

So, please bear with us, or skip ahead to chapter 2 (p. 27), as this section may not apply to everyone. But if it helps even one person feel more empowered, less confused or more in tune with their body, it has served its purpose.

Timing and frequency

The 'trying naturally' stage often brings a mix of hope, excitement and worry. You may feel unsure about timing, wonder whether you are doing things right or feel anxious each month as you wait to see what happens. All of that is normal. So, we are going to walk through this with you. We will talk about fertile windows, timing, signs to look for, common misconceptions and how to approach this stage without turning it into a source of stress or self-blame.

You know your body a little better now. Let's take that knowledge with us and explore what trying naturally can look like.

How often should you have sex?

People tend to overcomplicate this. The simplest, most evidence-based approach is as follows:

- Every two to three days throughout your menstrual cycle.
- Daily or every other day during your fertile window (*see* below).

Radical honesty: More-frequent sex does not harm sperm. Less-frequent sex does not create stronger sperm. This is about gentle consistency, not perfection.

Understanding your fertile window

As discussed earlier in the chapter (*see* pp. 19–20), pregnancy can happen during only a very small part of your menstrual cycle. Your fertile window includes the five days leading up to ovulation and the day of ovulation itself. Trying after ovulation is usually too late, and many people have simply never been told this.

The aim here is not to add pressure or turn timing into a rigid task but to help you understand your body's natural signals. We see people all the time who have been obsessing over timing, worrying that they are missing their fertile window or feeling terrified that they are doing everything wrong. This is completely natural when no one has explained things clearly before. Let's strip away the pressure and show you what actually matters.

When exactly should you try?

Your most fertile days are the days leading up to ovulation, not after. Your body gives you signals when that window is opening. The most reliable way to judge this is through working out when you may be ovulating. Here's how to track ovulation simply:

- Cervical mucus changes: Your cervical mucus becomes clear, slippery and stretchy, like raw egg whites. If it stretches into a long, stringy thread between your fingers, your fertile window is open.

- Ovulation predictor kits (OPKs): These look for your LH surge, which tells you that ovulation is likely 12–36 hours away. If your test turns positive, try that day and the next day.
- Apps: Apps are useful for logging menstrual cycles, but do not rely on them to predict ovulation. They work from averages, not your individual physiology.

Choose the method that feels easiest for you. If you prefer to keep things simple, watch for cervical mucus changes and try every two to three days throughout your cycle. If you like something more structured, use OPKs and have sex on the day the test turns positive and again the next day. If an app helps you log things, use it for awareness, not prediction.

The aim is not perfect timing. It is understanding your own signs well enough to give yourself the best chance without turning it into a source of pressure.

Basal body temperature: a more detailed way to track ovulation

If you would like a more detailed and data-driven way to track ovulation, basal body temperature (BBT) is one option. Identifying slight rises in temperature can help you predict when you are ovulating, giving you the best chance of conceiving naturally.

Steps to track BBT

Use a digital or mercury basal thermometer that measures to two decimal places (e.g., 36.52°C or 97.65°F).

Measure your BBT daily, at the same time each morning, immediately upon waking and before eating, drinking or moving. Record your readings and identify patterns. Over a few menstrual cycles, you'll notice a biphasic pattern:

- Lower temperatures before ovulation.
- Higher temperatures after ovulation.

How to time intercourse using BBT

Track your BBT for two to three menstrual cycles. Use the results to predict ovulation and identify your fertile window, which typically occurs two to three days before ovulation.

Plan intercourse during your fertile window. BBT confirms ovulation after it occurs, but sperm can survive up to five days in fertile cervical mucus. Timing intercourse in the days leading up to the temperature rise can maximise your chances.

Monitor the luteal phase. A sustained rise in BBT confirms ovulation. Tracking the length of your luteal phase (12–16 days) will help support conception.

Radical honesty: BBT is best at confirming ovulation has happened rather than predicting it in advance. For some people, this information is empowering. For others, it can feel like a lot of effort for something that's only clear in hindsight.

UNDERSTANDING YOUR BBT READINGS

- Preovulation (follicular phase): BBT is relatively low, typically ranging from 36.10–36.40°C (97.00–97.50°F). These lower temperatures are due to oestrogen, which dominates this phase.
- Ovulation: A slight drop in BBT may occur just before ovulation, but it's not always noticeable.
- Postovulation (luteal phase): After ovulation, rising progesterone causes a BBT increase of 0.30–0.50°C (0.50–1.00°F). This temperature shift confirms ovulation has occurred.
- Pregnancy: If conception happens, BBT remains elevated due to sustained progesterone production.
- No pregnancy: If conception does not occur, progesterone levels drop, causing a decrease in BBT and signalling the start of a new menstrual cycle.

Does position matter?

No. It really does not.

Sperm move far too quickly and efficiently for gravity or position to influence conception. You do not need to lift your legs, lie still afterwards, tilt your pelvis or stay in bed.

And listen, we will be honest. We have tried some of these things ourselves. When you want something so deeply, you will try anything that feels like it might help. But the science is clear: once ejaculation happens, sperm begin moving within seconds.

Use whatever position feels good and comfortable.

Radical honesty: Pleasure and connection matter. Pressure and performance do not.

A NOTE FOR PARTNERS WITH SPERM

Trying naturally is often framed as something that happens inside the woman's body, but sperm health is also shaped by timing and simple habits. One of the most helpful things a partner with sperm can do is maintain regular ejaculation.

Ejaculating every two to three days is ideal. Long gaps do not 'strengthen' sperm; in fact, they can increase the number of older, less-efficient sperm in the sample. Equally, ejaculating frequently does not harm sperm quality. The body is always making new sperm, and regular release simply supports that process.

This is not about schedules or performance. It is about a small, practical way of contributing that often gets overlooked.

If you do later move into treatment, clinics will usually ask for a two- to five-day abstinence window before you provide a sample, but outside of that context, gentle consistency is enough.

What not to panic about

Here are a few things that many people worry about but that often matter far less than they fear:

- Not seeing textbook 'egg-white' mucus every menstrual cycle.
- Missing a day, or even a few days, of trying.
- Your OPK not peaking on the same day each month.
- Menstrual cycles that are longer or shorter than 28 days.
- Sex feeling a bit pressured sometimes.
- A month where nothing feels predictable at all.

These things happen to almost everyone trying naturally. They do not mean something is wrong with you or your body.

It is easy to say, but try to hold in your mind that trying naturally is not about perfection. It is about working with your body rather than against it, learning its rhythms and letting go of the belief that you have to get every detail right. The more you understand your menstrual cycle, the less you need to rely on guesswork and the more grounded you can feel in the process. Take what is helpful from this section and leave the rest behind.

Above all, stay gentle with yourself. You are already doing more than you realise, simply by learning about and listening to your body in this way.

In summary

We have covered a lot in this chapter; our hope is that you now have a clearer understanding of the basics of your menstrual cycle, your hormones and what your body is trying to do each month. Before you move on, it might be helpful to pause for a moment and notice how all of this has made you feel. When you start tuning in to your body, it is just as important to start tuning in to your emotions too, because they are part of the same whole wonderful system that is you!

You might like to ask yourself gently: What has come up for me as I read this? Do I feel relieved, sad, angry, hopeful, confused or something else entirely? Has anything I believed about my body shifted, even slightly? Is there anything I would like to come back to, ask more about or speak to someone I trust about?

There are no right or wrong answers here. Whatever you feel is valid. Simply noticing your response is a way of honouring yourself and beginning this journey with honesty.

When you are ready, in the next chapter, we will begin to look at why pregnancy sometimes does not happen – even when you are doing all you can.

2

Understanding what might be getting in the way

One of the first questions many people ask when they begin struggling to conceive is, 'Why is this happening?' Or, if we are completely honest, 'Why is this happening to me?'

It is a question that deserves a clear and thoughtful response, and that is what this chapter is all about. The process of finding answers can be complex, but we will take you through the key things that may be influencing your fertility.

For some people, fertility difficulties can be identified quickly. A simple blood test, a routine scan or an early conversation with a healthcare professional may point to a clear cause. When this happens, there can be a sense of relief and direction. Understanding what is going on can help restore a feeling of control during a time that may feel unpredictable.

For many others, diagnosis takes much longer: sometimes months, sometimes years. This delay is not linked to anything they did or did not do; instead, it reflects the complexity of human reproduction. Fertility is influenced by an intricate mix of biology, genetics, medical history, hormones, lifestyle and, sometimes, chance. Because of this, discovering what is happening can take time, and that period of waiting can be one of the hardest parts of the journey.

If you are in that space where tests are inconclusive, where each appointment brings more questions than answers and where the path forwards feels uncertain, you may feel understandably stretched by the process. We understand the toll this takes.

We would love for you to remember this: you are not failing, you are not being overlooked and you are not alone.

For us, it goes without saying that no matter where you are in your journey – whether you have a diagnosis, are still searching for answers or are unsure where to begin – you deserve to feel seen, understood and supported. This chapter is here to offer guidance, reassurance and honesty. It is also here to remind you:

- You are allowed to ask questions.
- You are allowed to feel confused.
- You are allowed to hope.
- You are allowed to seek support at every step, especially when the answers come slowly or feel unclear.

With that in mind, it can help to begin by exploring some of the most common factors that may influence conception. Understanding these areas will not give you every answer, but it can offer a clearer sense of where difficulties sometimes arise. So, in this chapter, we will look at the areas where the process can break down and why conception doesn't always happen, even when you're doing everything 'right'.

It is entirely up to you how you use this chapter. Some people may want to read it from start to finish, while others will scan straight to the parts that feel most relevant. This is your journey, and you are allowed to use this book in whatever way helps you most.

Ovulation problems

One of the first places many clinics look is ovulation, since regular ovulation is essential for natural conception.

As we saw in the previous chapter, ovulation is the moment in each menstrual cycle when your ovary releases an egg (*see* p. 17). Once released, the egg is available for fertilisation for a short window, usually around 12–24 hours. If sperm are already present in the reproductive tract or arrive soon after ovulation, fertilisation can happen. If there are no sperm, the egg simply dissolves and the menstrual cycle continues as normal.

When ovulation is regular, it becomes easier to predict when this fertile window might occur. When ovulation is irregular or does not happen, the egg is released at unpredictable times or not released at all, respectively. This makes conception more difficult, because sperm and egg are less likely to meet at the right moment.

What this might look like for you

You may notice that your menstrual cycles are irregular, particularly long or short or sometimes absent. You may find that ovulation tests never give you a clear answer or that you get positives at unpredictable moments. For some people, the signs that point to different stages of the cycle (*see* pp. 19–20) appear inconsistently. This can make it more difficult to identify where you are in the cycle and therefore harder to identify your fertile window.

As mentioned in the previous chapter, people usually start assessing ovulation through an at-home OPK. However, many people assume that if the expected LH surge does not appear on an OPK, the body has not released an egg. This is not always the case.

Radical honesty: OPKs are less reliable than bloods and scans, but they are a good place to start.

CASE STUDY: ZARA – NO SURGE DETECTED

When Zara first started using ovulation tests, she expected them to guide her neatly through each menstrual cycle. She imagined she would see a clear positive every month and that this would confirm she was doing everything 'right'. Instead, the tests stayed negative again and again. After three cycles with no visible surge, Zara began to assume she was not ovulating at all. Each blank test strip felt like evidence that something was wrong.

By the time she spoke with her GP, Zara was preparing herself for difficult news. Her clinician suggested a blood test at the beginning of her period and in the middle of the luteal stage to see what was actually happening. The result showed that she had ovulated that month. The same happened the following cycle. In other words, ovulation had been occurring, but the tests had not captured it. The surge in LH had simply been brief, easy to miss and different in pattern to what the kits are designed to detect.

This changed the conversation entirely. Zara was not dealing with an absence of ovulation but with a tracking method that did not match the way her body signalled each month. Understanding this softened the sense of failure she had been carrying. It also helped her make decisions from a clearer and more grounded place.

Sometimes the difficulty comes from the way ovulation is being tested, and at other times ovulation itself may be irregular or disrupted.

What if you discover that you are not ovulating?

If your results from further investigations (such as blood tests and scans) show that ovulation is not happening, the next step is to understand why. This usually involves a few targeted tests that look at the hormones involved in ovulation and at how the ovaries are responding to these hormones (*see* pp. 66–72). From there, your clinician can talk through what the findings mean and what options are available.

In the rest of the chapter, we will explore the most common reasons that ovulation can be disrupted, what they mean for fertility and how each may be approached.

Polyendocrine metabolic ovarian syndrome (PMOS)

One of the most common reasons for disrupted ovulation is polyendocrine metabolic ovarian syndrome (PMOS), previously referred to as polycystic ovary syndrome (PCOS).

Not everyone with PMOS will experience fertility difficulties, and not everyone with irregular menstrual cycles has PMOS, but understanding this condition can help make sense of how and why ovulation sometimes becomes unpredictable.

PMOS is a hormonal condition that can affect ovulation, menstrual cycles and overall fertility. People often receive a diagnosis in different ways. Some have known about it for years. Others only hear the term for the first time when they begin trying to conceive. This section is for you whether you already have a diagnosis, think you may have PMOS or simply want to understand how it can play a role in fertility.

What PMOS may look like

PMOS tends to involve a combination of features. You may recognise some of the following:

- Irregular menstrual cycles: Periods may be infrequent, unpredictable or unusually long. This is often the most noticeable sign, and it makes ovulation difficult to track.
- Higher androgen levels: Androgens are sometimes called 'male hormones'. When they are raised, they can contribute to acne, oily skin or unwanted hair growth.

- Polycystic ovaries on ultrasound: An ultrasound may show many small follicles. These can give the ovaries a particular appearance, although this pattern does not confirm PMOS on its own.

Other common experiences: Some people with PMOS notice weight gain or difficulty losing weight, insulin resistance or thinning hair. Others have only one or two symptoms and may not realise they have PMOS until they begin fertility investigations.

If any of these features sound familiar, it may be helpful to discuss them with a clinician. There may be nothing wrong, but understanding your body and working out what may be going on for you as an individual can support more informed choices about your fertility and wellbeing.

Does having PMOS mean you will struggle to conceive?

Not necessarily. Many people with PMOS conceive naturally, without medical treatment. For others, PMOS affects how often ovulation happens, which can make conception less predictable. Support is available if ovulation is irregular or absent, and many people respond well to simple interventions.

Hypothalamic dysfunction

Not all ovulation difficulties come from the ovaries themselves. Sometimes, the reason sits a little higher up in the system, in the part of the brain that helps to regulate the menstrual cycle. When this area is under strain, the signals that guide ovulation can become quieter or less consistent. This is known as hypothalamic dysfunction, and it is one of the more subtle causes of irregular or absent ovulation.

The hypothalamus is a small but important part of the brain that sends hormonal signals to coordinate the menstrual cycle and ovulation. When the hypothalamus is under pressure, these signals can become weaker or less regular; this can lead to irregular or absent ovulation, even when the ovaries themselves are healthy.

The hypothalamus responds closely to the body's overall environment. Factors such as prolonged stress, very intense exercise, significant weight loss or gain, illness or a period of under-fuelling can all influence how it functions. These experiences may shift the body into a mode where reproduction is not prioritised, which in turn affects the hormones responsible for ovulation.

What this might look like

Some people notice their periods becoming lighter or less frequent, or stopping altogether. Others may see changes after a time of stress, heavy training or altered eating patterns. It is also possible to have no obvious symptoms other than difficulty predicting ovulation or conceiving.

CASE STUDY: POLLY – WHEN THE BODY IS UNDER STRAIN

Polly had always enjoyed being active. Movement was a core part of her life, and she found it grounding and energising. Over time, though, her training became more demanding. She was preparing for competitive events, fitting in long sessions most days and holding herself to a very strict routine around food and performance. None of this was intentional harm. It was simply the pattern she slipped into as her goals grew.

When Polly and her partner decided to try for a baby, she noticed her menstrual cycles were irregular. Some months, her period arrived later than expected. Other months, it did not come at all. Ovulation tests were inconsistent, and after several cycles of uncertainty, she asked her GP for advice. Blood tests suggested her body was not ovulating regularly, and she was referred for further assessment.

The specialist explained that her results were consistent with hypothalamic suppression. In simple terms, the part of the brain that sends the hormonal signal to begin ovulation had become quieter. The combination of intense training, low body fat for her frame and the day-to-day pressure she was living with had placed her body in a state it interpreted as strain. Under these conditions, some people temporarily stop ovulating as a protective response.

Hearing this was both surprising and relieving for Polly. She had not realised how much pressure she had been under or how finely tuned the reproductive system can be. With guidance, she made measured adjustments to her training load and nutrition. She also began paying attention to rest in a way she had not done before. Over time, her menstrual cycles returned and she started ovulating more regularly.

Exercise does not disrupt ovulation, and regular movement is one of the most supportive things you can do for your health. What affects the reproductive system is sustained physical strain, under-fuelling or a combination of intense training and everyday stress. When these pressures build, the brain may reduce or pause the signal that leads to ovulation. Understanding this is about clarity, not blame, and clarity allows for gentle and effective change.

What you can do now

If hypothalamic dysfunction is suspected, your clinician may look at the pattern of your menstrual cycle, your hormone levels and lifestyle factors (such as nutrition, stress levels, exercise and energy balance) to understand what is happening. Small, supportive changes to nutrition, stress, rest and exercise can often make a meaningful difference. You do not need to navigate these decisions alone. A clinician can help you identify the adjustments that are most relevant to your situation and plan next steps that feel manageable.

Again, addressing hypothalamic dysfunction is not about blaming you for any choices you have made. It is about creating conditions that allow your body to feel safe to ovulate again. Understanding the role of the hypothalamus can help you make sense of what your body is communicating and guide you towards a gentler, more supported approach to restoring hormonal balance.

As you can see, the signals that guide ovulation are sensitive to many aspects of health, including the way in which the body responds to stress, nourishment and physical demands. Hormones outside the reproductive system, including thyroid hormones, also play an important role.

Thyroid disorders

The thyroid, a small gland at the front of your neck, plays a surprisingly large role in fertility and how your body functions. It influences metabolism, energy levels, mood, menstrual cycles and ovulation. It also has an important role in early pregnancy. When it is underactive or overactive, it can affect ovulation in ways that are easy to overlook. Because its symptoms can be vague, thyroid issues often go unnoticed for years and are easily attributed to stress, tiredness or simply 'being busy'.

Thyroid conditions tend to fall into two broad groups: underactive and overactive thyroid. An underactive thyroid produces too little hormone. This is called hypothyroidism. An overactive thyroid produces too much hormone and is known as hyperthyroidism. Other people have an autoimmune thyroid condition, where the immune system affects the thyroid's ability to function. Hashimoto's and Graves' disease are examples of this.

These conditions can influence fertility in several ways. They can disrupt ovulation, alter the pattern of menstrual cycles and sometimes affect the quality of eggs or the development of the uterine lining. As thyroid hormones play a role in early pregnancy, undiagnosed or untreated thyroid problems can sometimes increase the risk of pregnancy loss or other complications.

What thyroid symptoms may look like

Thyroid symptoms vary widely. Some people notice changes in energy, weight, mood or hair. Others experience shifts in their menstrual cycle, or they simply have a sense that something is not quite right but cannot pinpoint why. Many people have no obvious symptoms at all until they begin trying to conceive and blood tests bring the issue to light.

THYROID HEALTH MATTERS FOR MEN, TOO

Thyroid hormones affect male fertility by influencing sperm production, sexual function and libido. Imbalances can reduce sperm count or movement, and can sometimes affect erectile function. For couples trying to conceive, it is often helpful to assess thyroid function in both partners.

How thyroid issues are investigated

Thyroid function is assessed through blood tests, which help clinicians understand not just whether the thyroid is being stimulated but also whether thyroid hormones are being produced.

Treatment of thyroid conditions

Most importantly, thyroid disorders respond well to treatment. Many people see improvements in their menstrual cycles and ovulation once thyroid hormone levels have been stabilised, and they go on to conceive naturally or with fertility support.

Radical honesty: Thyroid screening is sometimes overlooked in fertility assessments despite its importance. You do not need to

wait for clear symptoms or a long history of menstrual cycle changes to ask about your thyroid. A simple blood test can offer valuable information and prevent delays later in your fertility journey.

Low ovarian reserve

With thyroid health in mind, the next area to explore is ovarian reserve. This refers to the number of eggs remaining in the ovaries and how well those eggs are likely to respond to hormonal signals. Ovarian reserve does not define your chances of becoming pregnant, but it can provide useful context as you move forward, as it may influence fertility planning and treatment.

As we saw in chapter 1 (*see* p. 16), everyone is born with all the eggs they will ever have, and this number naturally declines with age. For some people, the decline happens more quickly than expected. When this happens, it is sometimes called low ovarian reserve.

Low ovarian reserve is not the same as menopause, and it does not mean pregnancy is impossible. It simply means there are fewer eggs available, which can influence how your body responds to treatment and how your fertility team plans the next steps.

What this might look like

Many people only learn about their ovarian reserve once they begin investigating their fertility. You may not notice any symptoms in daily life. Some people with low ovarian reserve continue to have regular periods; others have periods that become closer together. Some experience no changes at all. Low ovarian reserve is often discovered through blood tests or ultrasound rather than through how you feel.

How it is assessed

Ovarian reserve is usually assessed using a combination of blood tests and ultrasound findings. The results help clinicians understand how the ovaries are responding and can guide planning, but they do not predict whether pregnancy is possible. Because these tests can raise a lot of questions, we look at them in detail in chapter 3 (*see* pp. 66–72), where we explain what they measure and how the results are interpreted in context.

What you can do now

If you have been told you have a low ovarian reserve, the next step is to understand what the result means in the context of your age, your menstrual cycle, your medical history and your hopes. Your clinician may repeat the test, combine it with an ultrasound or talk through how the results might influence next steps.

Some people choose to move towards treatment sooner. Others pause to think, gather information or explore different routes to building a family. There is no single correct response, and you do not need to rush to a decision. Supportive options may include:

- A review of your full hormone profile.
- A discussion about the timing of trying to conceive (*see* pp. 21–23).
- Information about IVF stimulation strategies (*see* pp. 214–17).
- Exploring treatment add-ons (*see* chapter 9).
- Emotional and psychological support to help you manage the uncertainty that this kind of result can bring.

Radical honesty: Low ovarian reserve does not define your fertility. It is one piece of information, and it sits alongside many others. Understanding your ovarian reserve offers one part of the picture. It tells you something about the quantity of eggs available and how the ovaries may respond to treatment. What matters most is how you understand it, how you are supported through it and what choices you make from here.

Endometriosis and adenomyosis

Beyond egg numbers, the environment in which fertilisation and implantation take place also plays a role. This is where conditions such as endometriosis and adenomyosis become relevant. These conditions do not affect everyone, but when they are present, they can influence fertility in meaningful ways. In this section, we will look at what they are, how they are diagnosed and why they matter in the wider context of trying to conceive.

However, before we look at what these conditions are, it is important to acknowledge the lived experience behind them, especially if you have been living with symptoms for a long time without clear answers. Endometriosis and adenomyosis are not simply heavy periods. They are not normal period pain, and they are not something you need to tolerate because you have been told it is 'just part of being a woman'. These conditions can influence how you live, work and relate to others and shape your experience of your own body.

If you have been living with heavy bleeding, significant period pain, bowel or bladder symptoms, pelvic pressure, bloating, fatigue or a repeated sense that something is not right, it is understandable to want clarity. Many people with endometriosis or adenomyosis describe experiences of feeling unheard or unsure. Diagnosis can take years – across the world, the average time to diagnosis has been reported as seven to ten years – and those years often come with confusion, repeated appointments and advice that does not match lived experience.

While waiting for a diagnosis, people often learn to plan their days around symptoms or to mask pain so effectively that others assume they are coping. Some people live with symptoms throughout their menstrual cycle, not just during their period. Pain can occur during ovulation, during bowel movements, during sex or at unpredictable times. The effects of this can be wide-reaching, influencing relationships, work and emotional wellbeing.

There is an encouraging change happening. More people are speaking openly about these conditions. More clinicians are training in them. Public awareness is growing. Research is expanding. Slowly, the pathway to diagnosis and treatment is improving.

Before we move into the medical explanation, it may help to pause and recognise that living with these conditions often requires a level of strength and persistence that is rarely acknowledged.

What endometriosis and adenomyosis are

Endometriosis is a chronic condition where tissue similar to the lining of the uterus grows outside the uterus. It is most often found on the ovaries, fallopian tubes and pelvic structures, although it can appear in other areas. This tissue responds to hormonal changes and can cause inflammation, scar tissue and adhesions (*see* pp. 41–43).

Adenomyosis is a related condition where the same type of tissue grows into the muscle of the uterus itself. This can cause the uterus to become enlarged and can result in heavy, painful periods.

Both conditions vary widely. Some people have extensive disease and minimal symptoms. Others have significant symptoms with only small areas affected. Neither the severity of the pain nor the impact on fertility can be reliably predicted by the amount of tissue present.

Symptoms that may suggest endometriosis or adenomyosis

Symptoms differ from person to person, and some people may not have any symptoms at all. Common experiences include:

- Painful periods
- Pain during sex
- Chronic pelvic pain
- Heavy or prolonged bleeding
- Pain during bowel movements
- Bloating or pelvic pressure
- Difficulty conceiving

How these conditions may affect fertility

There are several ways in which endometriosis or adenomyosis can influence conception, but not all of them apply to everyone:

- Disrupted ovulation due to inflammation.
- Mechanical difficulties such as blocked or distorted fallopian tubes.
- Changes in the pelvic environment that affect egg and sperm interaction.
- Reduced egg quality or a lower ovarian reserve (*see* p. 35).
- Changes to how receptive the uterine lining is to an implanting embryo.

Radical honesty: If endometriosis is suspected and you are told it will not affect your fertility, it is reasonable to seek a second opinion. Endometriosis can influence egg quality, ovarian reserve, inflammation within the pelvis and the environment surrounding the egg and embryo. A fertility specialist and a gynaecologist often bring complementary perspectives, and seeing both can be helpful.

Adenomyosis – where tissue similar to the lining of the uterus grows within the muscular wall of the uterus, is also increasingly recognised as an important factor in fertility and pregnancy outcomes. It may contribute to painful periods, heavy bleeding, implantation difficulties, risk of pregnancy loss and challenges with embryo transfer or pregnancy maintenance. Although adenomyosis and endometriosis can occur separately, they commonly exist together, and both conditions deserve careful assessment as part of a full fertility work-up.

Approaches to management

Treatment is individual and usually aims to reduce symptoms, improve quality of life and protect or support fertility. Options may include medical management, surgical management, lifestyle considerations and assisted conception.

Medical management

Non-steroidal medicines can help manage pain. Hormonal treatments can reduce symptoms by suppressing the activity of the endometrial tissue, although they do not treat the underlying condition and may not be suitable if you are actively trying to conceive.

Surgical management

A laparoscopy can diagnose endometriosis and, in some cases, remove visible tissue. For some people, this can reduce pain and improve fertility outcomes, although surgery is not always necessary and decisions are best made with a specialist team.

Lifestyle considerations

For some people, dietary changes, gentle exercise and stress management can help support overall wellbeing. These are not treatments for endometriosis or adenomyosis, but they may ease some symptoms.

Assisted conception

If natural conception is proving difficult, assisted reproductive treatments such as IVF can help bypass some of the mechanical and inflammatory challenges associated with these conditions. This option does not treat endometriosis or adenomyosis but may improve the chance of pregnancy.

A NOTE ABOUT THE IMMUNE SYSTEM

Research suggests that endometriosis may involve changes in how the immune system behaves. These changes can influence inflammation, tissue growth and how the reproductive system functions. This does not mean that the immune system is overactive or dangerous. It simply reminds us that these conditions are complex and involve more than one body system. We explore immune-related factors in more detail later in this chapter (*see* pp. 52–53).

If endometriosis or adenomyosis is part of your picture

A diagnosis of endometriosis or adenomyosis can bring mixed feelings. For some people, it provides clarity. For others, it raises questions.

Whatever your experience, you do not need to navigate this alone. A specialist team can help you understand what your diagnosis means, what treatment options are available and what steps may support your fertility now and in the future.

Because these conditions often affect the structures in and around the pelvis, the next area we will explore is the fallopian tubes.

Blocked or damaged fallopian tubes

The fallopian tubes play a central role in natural conception, and understanding how they function can provide another piece of the wider fertility picture. These small structures provide the pathway for sperm to reach the egg, and they then carry the fertilised egg towards the uterus. When the fallopian tubes are blocked, scarred or not working as they should, this journey becomes harder. The egg may not be able to travel freely, and sperm may struggle to reach it. Even small areas of damage can interrupt these delicate passages.

Tubal problems can develop for several reasons. Some people have scarring after an infection or previous pelvic surgery. Others develop changes linked to endometriosis or pelvic inflammatory disease (PID). Whatever the cause, a blockage can prevent sperm and egg from meeting or stop a fertilised egg from travelling safely to the uterus. For some people, this reduces the chances of conceiving naturally.

What this might look like

Tubal issues often do not cause obvious symptoms. Many people discover there is a problem only when they begin investigating fertility. Some may recall a previous infection, surgery or severe pelvic pain, but for others there is no clear history. This can feel unsettling, especially when everything else appears normal. If this is where you find yourself, it is important to remember that tubal problems are common and can be assessed clearly with the right investigations.

How tubal health is assessed

If tubal factors are suspected, your clinician may suggest tests to check whether the fallopian tubes are open and functioning as they should. These assessments help clarify whether eggs and sperm are able to meet and whether a fertilised egg can travel safely to the uterus. Because these tests involve different techniques and experiences, we explain them in detail in chapter 3 (*see* pp. 64–65), where we walk through what each test involves and what the results can show.

When fallopian tubes are blocked or damaged, there is almost always a reason behind it. One of the most common causes is PID, a condition that can affect the tubes long before someone ever tries to conceive. Understanding how this happens can help you make sense of your own picture, especially if tubal changes have shown up unexpectedly in your tests.

Pelvic inflammatory disease (PID)

PID is an infection of the reproductive organs. It usually develops when bacteria travel from the vagina or cervix into the uterus, fallopian tubes or ovaries. In many cases, the bacteria are linked to sexually transmitted infections (STIs) such as chlamydia or gonorrhoea, although PID can also occur after childbirth, pregnancy loss or certain gynaecological procedures.

When the infection is treated early, many people recover fully. When it is not treated, inflammation can lead to scarring, narrowings or blockages inside the fallopian tubes. These changes can make it harder for sperm and egg to meet, and in some situations can increase the risk of an ectopic pregnancy (*see* pp. 46–47).

Radical honesty: One episode of PID can affect fertility. With several episodes, the risk becomes higher. This reflects the impact of repeated inflammation on the delicate structure of the fallopian tubes rather than anything about the person themselves.

Symptoms of PID vary widely. Some people experience pelvic pain, abnormal vaginal discharge, discomfort during sex or fever. Others have very mild symptoms or none at all, which can mean the infection goes unnoticed. This makes regular sexual health screening important if you are sexually active and at risk of STIs.

CASE STUDY – MARIA'S EXPERIENCE OF PID

Maria had her first pelvic infection in her early 20s. At the time, she was working long hours, sharing a busy flat and doing what many people do at that age: paying attention to some symptoms and hoping others would settle. When she noticed pelvic discomfort and a change in discharge, she assumed it was nothing serious. The symptoms came and went, and life moved on.

Over the next few years, she had two more episodes of what she now realises were likely infections. Each time, she felt unwell for a few days, then recovered. She did not know then that untreated infections can sometimes spread upwards in the pelvis and begin to cause inflammation around the fallopian tubes.

A decade later, when she and her partner began trying to conceive, things did not unfold as she expected. After several months of trying without success, her GP referred her for fertility investigations. When the results came back, the clinicians explained that both of her fallopian tubes showed signs of significant damage consistent with previous infection. The news was understandably hard to hear. Maria needed time to take in the idea that changes that had begun years earlier were now part of her present fertility story.

What made a difference was having the information explained clearly. Understanding that the damage was caused by infection and inflammation, not by something she had done or failed to do, created a sense of steadiness. It allowed her to focus on the next steps with a clearer mind. Her team talked her through the safest options for conception and helped her plan a route forwards that matched her situation.

What can help

If PID is diagnosed early, antibiotics can clear the infection and reduce the risk of long-term problems. Seeking medical attention as soon as symptoms begin is important, especially if you have pelvic pain, fever or unusual discharge. If the infection has been present for some time before treatment, there may be scarring or changes to the fallopian tubes. In this situation, your clinician can talk you through what the findings mean and what options are available to support conception. Even when damage has occurred, there are still clear routes forwards.

Protecting your reproductive health can feel complex, but there are some simple steps that can make a real difference. Regular STI screening if you are sexually active, using condoms when needed and seeking medical advice when something does not feel quite right are all practical ways to look after yourself. These are not judgements about behaviour. Many people do not realise they have had an infection at the time, and PID can develop quietly without dramatic symptoms.

Understanding the connection between untreated infections and future fertility can be confronting, especially if you are learning about it later. Awareness is not about blame. It is about giving yourself the information you need to make informed choices from this point forward.

Another area worth understanding relates to changes within the pelvis itself.

Adhesions

The next area to explore is the broader category of pelvic scarring and internal sticking known as adhesions, which can develop after infections, surgery or endometriosis and can also affect fertility.

You may hear your clinician mention adhesions. The word can sound worrying, so it might help to understand what it means. Adhesions are thin bands of scar tissue that form between organs or tissues after surgery, infection or inflammation. They are part of the body's healing process, but they can sometimes cause structures to stick together in ways that affect comfort or function.

When adhesions form in the pelvis, especially around the fallopian tubes or ovaries, they can change how these organs move or sit next to one another. In some situations, they can narrow or block a fallopian tube, or make it harder for the tube to pick up an egg after ovulation. This can reduce the chances of natural conception.

Previous abdominal or pelvic surgery can be a common reason for adhesions. Operations such as an appendicectomy, ovarian surgery or procedures for endometriosis all involve working close to the reproductive organs. As the body heals, the scar tissue that forms can sometimes create these internal sticky areas. The intention is protective, but the effect is not always helpful for fertility.

Radical honesty: Concerns about adhesions from previous surgery are sometimes minimised, yet they can be relevant. If you think this may apply to you, it is reasonable to ask your clinician to consider it carefully.

What can help

If your clinician suspects adhesions are affecting fertility, they may recommend imaging or, in some cases, a laparoscopy to understand what is happening. Surgery can sometimes release adhesions and improve the function of the fallopian tubes or ovaries, although this depends on where the adhesions are and how extensive they are. Your team will talk you through the benefits and limitations of your own diagnosis so you can make a decision that feels informed and manageable.

Adhesions are one example of structural changes that can influence fertility. The next step is to look at the uterus itself, since its shape, lining and overall health can all play important roles in conception and early pregnancy.

The uterus

When we hear that the uterus may be playing a role in our fertility, it can bring up many thoughts and questions. It is an intimate part of the body, and for many people it is tied to ideas about womanhood, identity and what it means to carry a pregnancy. Learning that something might be different or unexpected about your uterus can feel personal, even when the explanation is entirely anatomical.

Taking time to understand the structure of the uterus can help to turn something overwhelming into something more familiar and less intimidating. Your uterus has its own shape, history and story, and knowing more about it can help you make sense of what your clinicians are describing as you move through the fertility process.

Common uterine shapes and variations

Typical uterus

A pear-shaped uterus with a single cavity. This is the most common structure and usually supports pregnancy without difficulty.

Bicornuate uterus

A heart-shaped uterus with two upper cavities. This happens when the uterus does not fully fuse during development. It can be associated with a higher chance of pregnancy loss or preterm birth, although many people with a bicornuate uterus do carry healthy pregnancies.

Unicornuate uterus

A smaller uterus that develops from only one side. Conception is still possible, but this shape can influence implantation and increase the likelihood of complications in pregnancy.

Septate uterus

A band of tissue, known as a septum, divides the uterine cavity partially or completely. This can increase the risk of pregnancy loss because the septum has a different blood supply. Surgical removal of the septum can improve outcomes.

Arcuate uterus

A mild indentation at the top of the uterus. This is usually considered a normal variation and rarely affects fertility.

Didelphys uterus

Two separate uterine cavities, each with its own cervix. Pregnancy is still possible, but the structure may increase the chance of preterm birth or other complications.

T-shaped uterus

A narrow uterine cavity often linked to in-utero exposure to certain medications many decades ago. Some people with this shape experience difficulties conceiving or carrying a pregnancy.

Retroverted uterus

A uterus that tilts backwards rather than forwards. This is a common variation and usually has no impact on fertility. It can sometimes cause discomfort or be linked to other conditions, such as endometriosis.

CONGENITAL DIFFERENCES

Some uterine variations are present from birth and are noticed only during fertility investigations or following recurrent pregnancy loss (*see* pp. 47–48). These structural differences can influence how easily an embryo implants or whether the uterine cavity can stretch safely during pregnancy. Diagnosis usually involves imaging such as magnetic resonance imaging (MRI), ultrasound or hysterosalpingography (HSG).

Radical honesty: Concerns about uterine structure can be minimised, yet they are relevant for some people. If you think this may apply to

you, it is reasonable to ask your clinician to consider it carefully and to explain the findings in a way that makes sense to you.

How do I know what shape my uterus is?

Your clinician can assess the shape of your uterus using imaging. This is usually done with an ultrasound scan. In some situations, a more detailed picture is needed and a test such as hysterosalpingo contrast sonography (HyCoSy), hysteroscopy (*see* p. 199) or MRI may be recommended. These tests allow the clinician to see the outline of the uterine cavity, the thickness of the muscle and whether there are any features that might affect implantation or pregnancy.

Now that we have explored the role of the uterus in fertility, we can look at what happens when a pregnancy begins but does not progress in the usual way. The next section focuses on ectopic pregnancy and how it relates to the reproductive structures you have just read about.

Ectopic pregnancy

If you are reading this because you have experienced an ectopic pregnancy, we are sorry. An ectopic pregnancy is not only a medical event; it is a loss. It can arrive suddenly and bring fear, confusion and grief in equal measure. However other people may have described it to you, an ectopic pregnancy can be emotionally significant and deserves to be acknowledged as such.

An ectopic pregnancy happens when a fertilised egg implants outside the uterus, most often in a fallopian tube (*see* p. 14). In a typical pregnancy, the fertilised egg travels through the fallopian tube before settling into the lining of the uterus. When the journey is disrupted and implantation happens elsewhere, the growing tissue can stretch or rupture the tube. A pregnancy cannot grow safely in this position, and intervention is needed to protect your health. This is a medical emergency, and rapid care is essential.

Having an ectopic pregnancy can influence fertility in the future, mainly because of the possibility of damage to the fallopian tube on the affected side. The tube may become scarred, narrowed or blocked. This can make it harder for sperm to reach the egg or for a fertilised egg to move through the tube to the uterus. Some people go on to conceive naturally. Others may find that conception takes longer or need support from a fertility specialist.

Radical honesty: A previous ectopic pregnancy does increase the chance of another. This is not a certainty, but the risk is higher because structural changes to the fallopian tube can affect how future embryos travel.

What may help

If you have had an ectopic pregnancy, your medical team may suggest follow-up testing to understand the health of your remaining fallopian tube or tubes. This can include imaging to assess whether the tube is open. If there is significant damage, options such as IVF can offer an alternative route to pregnancy, because fertilisation takes place outside the body and embryos are placed directly into the uterus. This can reduce the chance of another ectopic pregnancy, although careful monitoring is still recommended.

Navigating the aftermath of an ectopic pregnancy takes time. There is no set pace. When you feel ready, a conversation with a fertility specialist can help clarify your current picture and the steps that may support you going forwards.

From here, we move to another part of the fertility picture that affects some people at a different stage of the journey. This is recurrent pregnancy loss, which sits alongside the other topics covered in this chapter as one of the recognised causes of difficulties conceiving or carrying a pregnancy.

Recurrent pregnancy loss

Recurrent pregnancy loss describes a situation where pregnancy ends without the birth of a live baby more than once, usually in the early stages. Different medical organisations define this slightly differently, with some defining recurrent pregnancy loss as two consecutive losses and others as three. Regardless of definitions, even a single pregnancy loss can carry enormous emotional weight and deserves recognition, support and appropriate medical care.

If this has been part of your story, it is important to recognise that pregnancy loss is not only a clinical issue but also a deeply personal experience. Each loss carries its own weight and meaning. Many people describe a mixture of shock, grief and uncertainty, and the question of why it keeps happening can feel heavy and unanswered. If this applies to you, please read this section with care for yourself, and pause whenever you need to.

There are many possible reasons why pregnancy does not continue, and most people need a careful and individual assessment to understand their own picture.

What may contribute to recurrent pregnancy loss

- Genetic factors: Sometimes, the embryo inherits a chromosomal difference that prevents further development (*see* pp. 49–51). This is one of the most common causes of early pregnancy loss.
- Hormonal imbalances: Certain hormonal patterns can affect how the uterine lining develops or how an early pregnancy is supported. This includes conditions where progesterone levels are not optimal.
- Structural differences: Variations in the shape of the uterus (*see* pp. 44–45) or the presence of fibroids (*see* pp. 65–66) or a septum can make implantation more difficult or increase the likelihood of early loss.
- Immune and clotting factors: Some autoimmune conditions, such as antiphospholipid syndrome, can affect blood flow to the developing pregnancy and increase the risk of pregnancy loss (*see* pp. 52–53).
- Lifestyle influences: Smoking, high alcohol intake and significant weight extremes can influence reproductive health. These factors are not causes on their own, but addressing them can support overall wellbeing and pregnancy outcomes.

The emotional impact

Repeated pregnancy loss can feel isolating, especially when the losses are early and invisible to others. Many people describe feeling caught between hope and fear with each new menstrual cycle. It may help to know that there is no correct way to respond emotionally. Your reaction is your own, and there is space for whatever you are feeling.

A recent development in the UK reflects a growing recognition of how significant early pregnancy loss is. As of March 2025, there is now statutory bereavement leave for pregnancy loss before 24 weeks, including miscarriage, ectopic pregnancy and molar pregnancy (a rare complication where abnormal fertilisation leads to the growth of abnormal tissue in the uterus instead of a healthy embryo and placenta). This change represents a small but meaningful step towards recognising that early loss deserves acknowledgement and support.

Radical honesty: Society often minimises early pregnancy loss and moves quickly to reassurance. This can leave people feeling unsupported or unseen. Recurrent pregnancy loss deserves careful investigation, clear information and emotional space.

How recurrent pregnancy loss is assessed

Your clinician will usually begin with a full medical history and then arrange a set of investigations. These may include the following:

- Blood tests to assess hormones and immune factors.
- Genetic testing for you and your partner.
- Imaging to examine the uterus and endometrial cavity.
- Further tests depending on your history.

This process takes time, but it helps build a clearer understanding of what might be happening.

What may help

If an underlying cause is identified, treatment can be tailored to address it. This may involve hormonal support in early pregnancy, a small surgical procedure to correct a uterine variation, treatment to reduce immune or clotting factors or lifestyle adjustments that support overall health.

Some people may be offered assisted conception with preimplantation genetic testing (*see* pp. 203–6) to help select embryos without chromosomal differences.

Emotional support can be equally important. Counselling, specialist miscarriage charities and support groups can provide connection, language and space to process what you have been through. Many people go on to have a healthy pregnancy after recurrent losses, but it is understandable if this feels hard to hold on to while you are still searching for answers.

From here, we look at one of the genetic factors that can influence both conception and pregnancy loss. This is chromosomal translocations, a less common but important area to understand in the wider picture of fertility.

Chromosomal translocations: understanding genetic rearrangements in fertility

Chromosomal translocations are changes in the structure of chromosomes. They occur when a segment of one chromosome breaks away and attaches to another, or when two chromosomes exchange pieces. Many people who carry a translocation are completely unaware of it. It often comes to light only during fertility investigations, after recurrent pregnancy loss or following the birth of a child with a chromosomal condition.

In a balanced translocation, no genetic material is missing or gained; it is simply arranged differently. Most people with a balanced translocation have typical health and no symptoms in everyday life. Where this difference can matter is during the formation of eggs or sperm. When chromosomes are passed on, some embryos may receive the correct amount of genetic material, while others may have extra or missing pieces. This can lead to early pregnancy loss, implantation difficulties or, more rarely, the possibility of having a child with a chromosomal or genetic condition.

These possibilities can feel unsettling, especially when this information is new. But understanding what is happening at a genetic level often brings clarity and helps you make decisions from a more grounded place.

How chromosomal translocations are identified

Translocations are usually detected through a blood test called a karyotype. This test looks at the number and structure of your chromosomes and can show whether a balanced translocation or other structural change is present.

If a translocation is found, your clinician may suggest that your partner is tested as well. Understanding who carries the rearrangement, and how it behaves genetically, helps guide treatment decisions and estimate the chances of different outcomes in future pregnancies.

What support may look like

If a translocation is identified, there are still meaningful paths forwards. Your medical team may talk with you about options such as IVF with preimplantation genetic testing for structural rearrangements (PGT-SR). This allows embryos to be screened for chromosomal balance before they are transferred to the uterus. Some people choose this route; others prefer to try naturally. Both are valid choices.

You may also be referred to a genetic counsellor. Their role is to explain the findings in a way that feels manageable, answer questions and help you understand what the results mean for you, your future pregnancies and, sometimes, for wider family members. Many people find these conversations reassuring, as they turn something that may feel abstract into a clearer and more navigable picture.

Other genetic factors

Chromosomal translocations are only one part of the wider genetic landscape. Other genetic conditions can also influence fertility or pregnancy outcomes in different ways.

Single-gene conditions

These occur when a change in one specific gene affects how the body functions. Examples include conditions such as cystic fibrosis, some forms of thalassaemia and conditions related to fragile X syndrome. Some of these affect reproductive health directly, while others mainly impact the health of future children.

Carrier testing can show whether you or your partner carry certain gene changes. If both partners carry the same recessive condition (*see* p. 76), there is usually a one in four chance in each pregnancy that a child will inherit it. Your team may then discuss options such as PGT-M (genetic testing for single-gene conditions), donor eggs or sperm or other pathways. These conversations should take place at a pace that feels safe for you.

Complex or polygenic traits

Some fertility-related traits, such as ovarian reserve or sperm production, are influenced by many genes working together, alongside environmental and lifestyle factors. These are called complex or polygenic traits. No single test can diagnose them, but your clinician may explain when genetics could be one contributing factor among several.

When family structure and background matter

In some cultures and families, marriages between relatives are traditional. This makes it more likely that both partners carry the same inherited gene change. If this applies to you, it is completely reasonable to ask about genetic screening, carrier testing or a referral to a genetic counsellor. The aim is not to create worry but to give you clarity so you can make informed decisions.

Bringing it all together

Genetic findings can feel complex and, at times, overwhelming. But they are only one part of the overall fertility picture. Genetic testing does not remove your chances of becoming a parent. Used well, it helps clarify risks, guide treatment choices and support planning for the future.

Many people with genetic findings, including balanced translocations or carrier status for single-gene conditions, go on to have healthy pregnancies and healthy children, either naturally or with treatment.

With the right information, supportive clinicians and time to process what you have learned, you can move forward in a way that honours both your emotions and your hopes.

From here, we move into an area that can feel less familiar and is often subject to mixed messages: the role of the immune system in fertility. While the science is evolving and not everything is fully understood, it is an important part of the wider picture for some people. Let's look at what is known in a clear and grounded way.

Immunological factors

The immune system is designed to protect you, but sometimes it becomes involved in fertility in unexpected ways. This happens when parts of the immune response begin to affect ovulation, implantation or the early stages of pregnancy. Immunological factors are not the most common cause of fertility difficulties, but when they are present, understanding them can make sense of a previously confusing picture.

Some immune-related conditions are already well known, such as systemic lupus erythematosus or rheumatoid arthritis. Others sit more quietly in the background until testing is done. For some people, the immune system may influence ovarian function, hormone balance or the uterine environment in ways that make conception and early pregnancy more difficult.

How the immune system can affect fertility

For implantation to occur, the immune system needs to recognise the embryo as something to welcome rather than something to reject. This requires a delicate balance. If the immune response is overactive, the embryo may struggle to implant. If it is underactive, inflammation may persist in ways that disrupt ovarian or uterine function.

Chronic inflammation can also make conception more difficult. This can happen in conditions such as endometriosis or PID, where inflammation in the pelvis affects eggs, sperm or the lining of the uterus. In autoimmune conditions, the immune system may mistakenly target tissues that play a role in early pregnancy.

Antiphospholipid syndrome

Antiphospholipid syndrome is an autoimmune condition in which the body produces antibodies that increase the tendency for blood to clot.

In fertility care, it is most closely associated with recurrent pregnancy loss. This is because small blood clots can affect the early placenta, reducing blood flow to the developing pregnancy. Diagnosis is made through blood tests that look for specific antiphospholipid antibodies.

Other immune factors

Some clinicians believe that other parts of the immune system play a role. This can include unusually high or low natural killer cell activity, an imbalance in cytokines (the signalling molecules that help regulate inflammation) or difficulties developing immune tolerance to an embryo. These areas are still evolving in terms of research and practice. When testing is recommended, it is usually done with specialist guidance.

Supporting fertility when the immune system is involved

Support varies depending on the diagnosis and who is treating you. For some people, managing an existing autoimmune condition is the most crucial step. This may involve medication, regular monitoring and working closely with both a fertility specialist and a rheumatologist or immunologist.

If a condition such as antiphospholipid syndrome is present, your team may recommend blood thinners or other treatments to reduce the risk of pregnancy loss. Close monitoring during early pregnancy is usually recommended. When other immune factors are suspected, your clinician may discuss whether additional testing or specialist input could be helpful.

From here, we move towards a part of the fertility picture that involves the other half of conception: the role of male factors, which can contribute to fertility challenges just as significantly as those on the female side.

The male factor

We have not explored male fertility in depth yet, but we are not overlooking it – chapter 4 is dedicated to this topic. For now, we will look briefly at how male factors fit into the wider picture of fertility.

If you are reading this as part of a couple, it may help to know that male factor fertility issues (such as low sperm count, reduced movement of sperm or a higher proportion of abnormally shaped sperm) are just as common a contributor to difficulties conceiving as female factor issues. Despite this, fertility is still often framed as something that belongs to women, which means many people are unaware of how significant sperm health really is. In addition, fertility investigations and treatments still predominantly take place in women's bodies. Even when the primary diagnosis is male factor, it is usually the woman who undergoes hormonal treatment, menstrual cycle monitoring and invasive procedures. This is one of the reasons much of this book focuses on women's health and experience while also making space to address male fertility clearly and directly.

What semen analysis involves

A semen analysis looks at sperm count, movement and shape, all of which can influence the likelihood of fertilisation. The results can be affected by a wide range of factors, including health, lifestyle and environment; sometimes, there is no clear cause at all. If the results raise concerns, support may include lifestyle changes, medical treatment or assisted reproduction, alongside emotional support for individuals and couples (*see* chapter 4 for a more in-depth look at male factor fertility, testing and next steps).

Sperm DNA Fragmentation

The Hidden Factor. Sometimes, sperm appears healthy under a microscope but carries unseen damage in its DNA. High DNA fragmentation can lead to lower fertilisation rates, poor embryo quality, and pregnancy loss.

Difficulty conceiving or carrying a pregnancy after previously having a child

We must now discuss one of the most important and often misunderstood areas of fertility care. This is secondary infertility, or the experience of having difficulty conceiving or carrying a pregnancy after previously having a child. Many people assume that if conception happened once, it will happen again in a similar way. When it does not, the experience can bring a mix of practical questions and emotional uncertainty.

Secondary fertility difficulties are common. In fact, a large proportion of fertility assessments in the UK involve people who have conceived before and are now finding it harder to do so.

Reasons for secondary infertility

There are many reasons why secondary infertility can happen. Some overlap with the causes already explored in this chapter, while others emerge over time.

Common factors include:

- Age: Fertility naturally declines with age. For some people, this becomes noticeable only when trying for a second child.
- Changes in reproductive health: Conditions such as endometriosis (*see* pp. 36–39), PMOS (*see* pp. 30–31) or hormonal shifts (*see* pp. 16–18) can develop or worsen over time.
- Immune factors: In some cases, the immune system can influence implantation or early pregnancy, making conception less predictable (*see* pp. 52–53).
- Experiences during previous pregnancy or birth: Complications, infections or procedures during or after a previous pregnancy can sometimes affect future fertility.
- Male factors: Sperm quality and quantity can change with time and may be influenced by age, underlying health conditions, past infections or hormonal factors (*see* chapter 4).

Diagnosis and treatment

If you are finding it harder to conceive again, the first step is a full assessment for both partners. This typically includes checking ovulation, a semen analysis and imaging to look for any structural changes or conditions that may have developed since the first pregnancy. Treatment will depend on what is found and may include:

- Medication to support ovulation or manage hormonal changes.
- Surgery if a structural issue is identified, such as a blocked fallopian tube or fibroid.
- Assisted conception treatments, including IVF, if these offer the most reliable route.
- In some cases, a discussion about other pathways to parenthood if needed, including surrogacy (*see* pp. 191–94) or adoption (*see* pp. 194–96).

Support at this stage is essential. Secondary fertility difficulties can bring a particular type of emotional complexity, because you may be balancing gratitude for the child you have with longing for another. Both experiences can sit side by side, and both are valid.

However, not every fertility story comes with a clear diagnosis. In the final part of this chapter, we will discuss unexplained infertility, which speaks to the experience of having normal test results and still finding conception difficult.

Unexplained infertility: making sense of things when medicine cannot

Being told you have unexplained infertility can feel deeply confusing. It is not a diagnosis in the traditional sense, as it does not tell you what is wrong. Instead, it means that even after a thorough assessment of hormones, ultrasound scans, tubal checks and semen analysis, there is no single identifiable reason to explain why conceiving has been difficult.

Unexplained infertility is surprisingly common. In the UK, around one-third of people seeking fertility care receive this explanation. It can be unsettling, because many of us feel safer when we have something concrete to work with. When we face a problem, we want a cause, a label, something that points to a clear solution. Yet unexplained infertility sits in a quieter place. It tells you that nothing obvious has been found, even though conception has not happened.

It is important to remember that 'unexplained' does not mean 'untreatable'. Instead, it means that the standard tests have not shown a clear reason. Human reproduction is complex, and current medical tests cannot capture every element of it. Hormones fluctuate subtly. The immune system interacts with implantation in ways that are not fully understood. Egg and sperm compatibility cannot always be measured. Even emotional and psychological factors can influence the hormonal rhythms that support reproduction.

None of these possibilities suggest that your body is failing. They mean that your body's story does not fit neatly into the categories medicine currently has.

Radical honesty: Society often responds to unexplained infertility with well-meaning phrases such as, 'Relax and it will happen' or 'Give it time'. These comments can feel minimising. When there is no clear explanation, many people understandably turn inwards and wonder if they have missed something or caused something. You may find thoughts like, *There must be something wrong with me* rising quietly in the background. These thoughts are common but not necessarily true.

Many people with unexplained infertility do eventually conceive, with or without treatment. Others build their families through different, equally meaningful routes. Progress is still possible, even when clarity is not.

What can help

Even without a clear 'why', there are still practical ways to move forwards. Some people choose timed sexual intercourse or ovulation support. Others explore fertility treatments such as intrauterine insemination (IUI) or IVF, which can bypass some unknown variables and increase the chances of fertilisation and implantation. These decisions do not need to be made quickly, and we will go through each of the treatment options in chapter 8. The most important step is understanding the options that feel right for you.

Emotional support can also make a difference. Psychotherapy, mind–body approaches, relationship support and stress management strategies are not about suggesting the cause is your fault. You deserve care that recognises your story, not just your test results. You deserve conversations where you feel heard, not dismissed.

CASE STUDY: PRIYA AND ALEX – NO KNOWN CAUSE

Priya, 32, and Alex, 35, had been trying to conceive for over two years. They both lived healthy lives and had no known medical issues. Priya's menstrual cycles were regular. After a year of trying, they saw a fertility specialist. Priya's hormone tests, ultrasound scans and tubal checks were all normal. Alex's semen analysis also fell within the expected range. With no clear explanation, they were given the diagnosis of 'unexplained infertility'.

The uncertainty was difficult for them. Priya found herself wondering whether she had somehow caused the problem. Alex felt frustration rising when every test came back normal. They decided to seek counselling to help them understand the emotional strain and to strengthen their communication. They continued to explore fertility options at a pace that felt manageable, while keeping a focus on their overall wellbeing.

Our reflection

Unexplained infertility invites us into a space that medicine is still learning to understand. It reminds us that not every part of human reproduction is visible on a scan or measurable in a blood test. It reminds us that science, as advanced as it is, has limits. When there is no explanation, the default assumption for many people is that the explanation must lie within themselves. This is an understandable but painful leap. However, the absence of an answer does not mean the answer is you.

Sometimes, the truth is simply that biology is complex, and current knowledge has not yet caught up with your particular story. Your body is not a problem to be solved. It is a system with layers of subtlety that science is still unravelling.

Unexplained infertility does not take away your potential for having a child. It places you in a part of the fertility landscape where the path is less mapped. Your journey may not be linear, but it remains yours, and you are not moving through it alone.

Final thoughts

As we have seen in this chapter, there are many reasons why conceiving can be difficult, and those reasons can be complex, overlapping and deeply individual. You may recognise one clear factor in your own story, or you may conclude that more than one area could be involved. Fertility is rarely shaped by a single explanation. It is influenced by biology, circumstance, timing, relationships and the emotional landscape in which all of this unfolds.

If you are reading this while trying to understand what might be happening for you, it may help to remember that fertility is not only a medical experience. It is also a psychological and relational one. The process can ask a great deal of you, and it is understandable to want to seek clarity, direction and reassurance along the way. Speaking with healthcare professionals, accessing counselling or connecting with others who have faced similar uncertainty can bring steadiness when the path ahead feels unclear.

As you move forwards, try to hold your situation with compassion and patience. Being informed gives you choices. Having support gives you strength. And staying connected to what matters to you can help you navigate this experience in a way that feels grounded and authentic.

Now that we have explored the main factors that can affect conception, it may help to take a step forwards and look at fertility tests (and specifically blood and hormone tests) more closely. The next chapter will guide you through each test in clear, simple language so you can understand what your results are showing and how they fit into the wider picture of your fertility.

3

When to test, and what your fertility tests really mean

There comes a moment in many people's fertility journeys when questions begin to surface: *Should I wait a little longer? Should I ask for help? Am I worrying too soon? Am I waiting too long?*

This chapter is here to offer clarity, without predictions or pressure. It shares clear, grounded information about when it may be helpful to consider fertility testing, how the process usually begins, and what the tests themselves are looking for and may mean for you.

Everything is broken down gently, with no assumption of medical knowledge. You do not need to learn every term or hold all of this in your mind at once. Think of this chapter as something you can return to whenever you need a little more light on what is happening.

We will begin by looking at when it may be helpful to consider fertility testing.

When to consider testing

There are some broad guidelines in the UK that can help you decide when it may be time to seek advice:

- If you are under 35, it is generally recommended to consider seeking advice after 12 months of trying.
- If you are between 35 and 39, it may be helpful to seek advice after 6 months.
- If you are 40 or older, it is sensible to speak to a specialist earlier rather than later.

These timelines exist because egg quantity and quality change with age, and we believe that earlier planning can help protect your options.

You may also want to consider requesting testing sooner if any of the following apply:

- Your periods are irregular or absent.
- Your periods are very painful or interfere with daily life.
- You have PMOS (*see* pp. 30–31) or endometriosis (*see* pp. 36–39).
- You have had two or more miscarriages (*see* pp. 47–48).
- You have had pelvic surgery or cancer treatment.
- Your partner has known sperm concerns (*see* pp. 86–88) or ejaculation difficulties (*see* p. 92).

These situations do not automatically mean that something is wrong. They are signals that testing may offer useful clarity earlier, rather than leaving you in uncertainty.

> **Radical honesty: Ovarian ageing is real. Egg quantity and quality do change over time. Lifestyle choices can support general health and may help egg and sperm quality, but they cannot stop ovarian ageing. This is biology, and it sits outside our control. Knowing this is not meant to scare you, even though it can sound daunting. It is intended to help you plan with both eyes open, rather than looking back wishing you had known sooner.**

And while we are talking about timing and planning, it is important to remember that fertility is not only about eggs. Male factor fertility matters, too. Around half of fertility challenges involve sperm, which is why both partners are usually tested early. In this chapter, we focus on understanding female fertility; male fertility and sperm testing are explored in chapter 4.

With all of this in mind, the next question is often a very practical one: where do you actually begin?

How to begin the testing process

In the UK, fertility testing usually begins when you request an assessment through your GP or a specialist fertility clinic. You do not need a rehearsed speech or the perfect wording. You can simply say, 'We have been trying to conceive for this many months and would like to begin a fertility assessment.' That is enough.

Before your appointment, it can help to jot down a few gentle notes. Nothing formal, just the key things you think might matter, such as:

- Your menstrual cycle pattern (for example, whether your cycles are regular or irregular, their average length and any changes you have noticed over time).
- Any pregnancies or losses.
- Any long-term conditions or abdominal/ gynaecological surgeries.
- Any lifestyle factors you feel may be relevant (such as smoking, alcohol intake, exercise patterns, stress levels or sleep).
- How long you have been trying.

These details help your doctor understand the wider picture without you needing to remember everything on the spot.

At the appointment, it is reasonable to ask for clarity. For example, you can ask:

- What tests will be done.
- When the results will be ready.
- How you will receive the results.
- When you will be able to speak to someone who can explain what they mean.

Once you have taken this first step, the next question is often what happens next.

What testing usually involves

Early fertility testing is designed to give a basic picture of how your reproductive system is working. For women, this often includes:

- Blood tests to look at hormones.
- An ultrasound to examine the ovaries and uterus.
- A test to check whether the fallopian tubes are open, if needed.

For male partners, this usually involves a semen analysis (*see* pp. 83–86). Sperm results can change over time, so a second test is common if the first result looks unusual. And as we say, we take an in-depth look at the male factor in chapter 4.

It can be helpful to remember that no single result tells the whole story. Fertility is a pattern, not a moment. Once this initial assessment is complete, your doctor or clinic will usually have a clearer sense of whether further testing is needed and, if so, which tests will be most relevant.

In the rest of this chapter, we will walk through the fertility tests you are most likely to hear about, explaining what each one looks for and how results are generally interpreted. We will begin with ultrasound scans and hormone testing, as these are commonly part of early assessment.

Understanding the tests

Some tests look at structure (the health and physical condition of your reproductive organs), others look at hormones and some are only offered if earlier tests suggest a closer look would be helpful. You may not need every test described here. The aim is to help you recognise the names, understand what each test is used for and know what questions to ask if they are offered to you.

Ultrasound scan

An ultrasound scan is often one of the first and most useful fertility tests. It allows your clinician to look at your uterus and ovaries in real time and build an initial picture of how things look structurally.

You may be asked to have this scan while you are having your period or in the very early days of your menstrual cycle. This can feel surprising, but it is completely normal and is often the best time for clinicians to get clear, useful information.

Most fertility ultrasounds are performed internally using a small vaginal probe. This can sound intimidating, especially if you have never had one before, but it is usually gentle, quick and no more uncomfortable than a cervical smear. Here's what the ultrasound is looking for:

- The shape and structure of the uterus.
- The thickness of the uterine lining.
- The presence of fibroids or polyps (*see* pp. 65–66).
- The appearance of the ovaries.
- The number of small resting follicles in each ovary.

- Any signs of cysts or patterns associated with conditions such as PMOS (*see* pp. 30–31) or endometriosis/adenomyosis (*see* pp. 36–39).

The scan results are usually interpreted by looking at a few common features. Each one offers different information about fertility and helps guide what, if anything, needs further attention.

Typical findings and what they may mean

Uterus

A healthy uterus usually appears smooth and well shaped. This is simply a visual description, not a judgement.

The lining of the uterus naturally changes thickness across the menstrual cycle. Early in the cycle, it is thin, often around 2–5mm. As ovulation approaches and the body prepares for the possibility of pregnancy, the lining becomes thicker. Seeing this natural change is usually a reassuring sign that the uterus is responding to the menstrual cycle as expected.

Ovaries

Each ovary contains small fluid-filled sacs called follicles. These follicles hold the eggs that develop during the menstrual cycle. The ovaries are assessed for both follicle count and the presence of any cysts or swelling, as discussed below.

Antral follicle count

The antral follicle count (also referred to as AFC) refers to the number of small, resting follicles seen on each ovary during the scan. This is usually measured early in the menstrual cycle and is one of the ways in which clinicians estimate ovarian reserve:

- A combined count of around 10–25 follicles across both ovaries is often considered within the expected range for fertility.
- Lower numbers may suggest a reduced ovarian reserve.
- Higher numbers can reflect a pattern commonly seen in PMOS (*see* pp. 30–31).

It can help to know that this number is never interpreted on its own. Your AFC is one piece of information about how the ovaries are functioning, and it is usually considered alongside your age, hormone results and menstrual cycle history.

It is also worth holding in mind that follicle numbers change naturally with age and vary from person to person. For most people, the most useful question is not the number itself but what it means for you, in your particular situation.

Presence of cysts or swelling

Cysts or other changes in the ovaries might influence ovulation or the environment for conception.

Small, simple cysts are very common and are often part of how the ovaries behave across the menstrual cycle. They are usually harmless and resolve without any treatment.

Occasionally, a larger cyst or one with particular features may need to be monitored or assessed more closely. This does not automatically mean that something is wrong. More often, it means your clinician will keep an eye on it, repeat the scan at another point in your cycle or suggest further checks if they would be helpful.

Once the scan has helped build a picture of the uterus and ovaries themselves, the next question is sometimes whether the fallopian tubes are open.

Fallopian tube assessment

An ultrasound on its own cannot usually show whether the fallopian tubes are open. If your clinician needs this information, you may be offered a test such as an HSG, HyCoSy or laparoscopy.

An HSG is an X-ray test that uses a small amount of dye passed through the cervix into the uterus via a thin catheter. As the dye moves through the uterus and the fallopian tubes, the images show whether the tubes are open or blocked. The test is usually brief, and you will be awake throughout.

Some clinics use an ultrasound version of this assessment called a HyCoSy. If the fluid travels through the fallopian tubes and into the pelvis, this suggests that the tubes are open. Ultrasound is a gentler alternative to an X-ray for some people.

These procedures are usually performed while you are awake and can cause some cramping or discomfort, similar to period pain. Many people find it helpful to know in advance that this sensation is temporary and settles quickly.

In some situations, your clinician may recommend a laparoscopy. This is a keyhole procedure that uses a small camera to look directly at the pelvis, ovaries and fallopian tubes. It can help diagnose certain conditions and, in some cases, allow treatment at the same time. The procedure is usually performed under sedation or a light anaesthetic so that you are comfortable throughout. Most people go home the same day.

Tubal tests focus on whether eggs and sperm are able to meet. Once that pathway has been assessed, attention often shifts to the space where an embryo would need to settle and grow. A key consideration is whether anything there could make implantation more difficult, such as a polyp.

Polyps

Polyps are different from fallopian tube findings. They are small, soft areas of tissue that sit on the lining of the uterus itself. They can vary in size, from just a few millimetres to a couple of centimetres, and are often picked up during an ultrasound or hysteroscopy.

Most polyps are benign, and many people never know they have one unless it appears on a scan. Hearing that something has been found can feel unsettling, even when it is common, so it can help to know that polyps are a familiar and usually straightforward finding in fertility care.

Why they matter

Polyps can sometimes affect implantation because they slightly change the surface of the uterine lining. A small polyp may not cause any difficulty at all. However, a larger polyp, or one positioned near the centre of the uterine cavity or close to the opening of a fallopian tube, may reduce the chance of an embryo settling.

If a polyp is found, your clinician may suggest removing it. This is usually done through a simple procedure called a hysteroscopy, where the polyp is gently removed through the cervix, without any cuts to the abdomen. Although the word 'growth' can sound alarming, polyps are almost always benign and very treatable. This is also true for fibroids.

Fibroids

Fibroids are different from polyps. They are firm growths made of muscle and fibrous tissue that develop within the wall of the uterus. Fibroids can vary widely in size, from very small nodules that are only visible on a scan to larger growths that can change the shape of the uterus.

They can sit in different parts of the uterus. Some grow within the muscle of the uterine wall, some sit on the outer surface of the uterus, and others develop just beneath the lining of the uterus where a pregnancy would normally implant.

Fibroids are extremely common. Many people have them without ever knowing, and they are often discovered incidentally during a scan.

> **Radical honesty: Hearing that a fibroid has been found can feel worrying, but in many cases they cause no symptoms and do not interfere with fertility.**

Why they matter

Fibroids can sometimes affect fertility depending on their size and location. What matters most is whether the fibroid is changing the shape of the uterine cavity, the space where an embryo needs to implant and grow.

A fibroid sitting on the outside of the uterus, or small ones embedded within the muscle wall, often make little difference to fertility. However, a fibroid that pushes into the uterine cavity can alter the shape of that space or affect the uterine lining, which may make implantation more difficult.

> **Radical honesty: If a fibroid appears to be affecting the uterine cavity, your clinician may suggest removing it before treatment. This is usually done through a surgical procedure designed to restore the normal shape of the uterus. While hearing the word fibroid can feel unsettling, most are benign and many never require treatment at all.**

Once this part of the picture has been explored, attention often turns to another important area of fertility testing: how your menstrual cycle is being guided by hormones.

Hormone tests

Hormones are the body's messengers. They help your brain and your ovaries communicate with each other. When clinicians test hormones, they are trying to understand how smoothly that communication is working and whether ovulation is likely to be taking place.

Hormone levels can be influenced by many everyday factors, including stress, sleep, illness, the day of your menstrual cycle and even the time of day. It can help to think of them not as rigid facts but as indicators or starting points for understanding what is happening.

Below is an overview of the hormones and related tests you are most likely to come across, as well as what they are generally used to assess. You do not need to memorise any of this; instead, the aim is to help you recognise the names and understand the kind of question each test is trying to answer.

Anti-Müllerian hormone (AMH)

AMH provides an estimate of how many eggs you may have remaining. It does not tell you whether those eggs are healthy, and it does not predict whether you will get pregnant. It can help to think of AMH as information about quantity rather than quality.

AMH is often considered within the expected range when it is above around 7–8pmol per litre. Levels between 3 and 7pmol per litre are usually described as low, and levels below 3pmol per litre as very low. These thresholds vary between clinics, and AMH naturally declines with age.

One helpful way to consider AMH is as one piece of a much larger picture. It is usually interpreted alongside your age, ultrasound findings and often your FSH, rather than being used on its own.

Radical honesty: It can be difficult to hear that you have low AMH. Please know that it is not a verdict. It is a guide, and knowing sooner can give you time to make informed choices rather than sitting with uncertainty.

Follicle-stimulating hormone (FSH)

FSH helps your ovaries grow eggs each month. It is usually tested at the start of your menstrual cycle and gives clinicians a sense of how hard your brain is working to stimulate the ovaries. If the ovaries are less responsive, FSH can rise as the body tries to compensate.

An FSH level below 9IU per litre measured between day two and day five of the menstrual cycle is often considered within the expected range. Levels between 10 and 12IU per litre may suggest a reduced ovarian reserve. Levels above 12IU per litre can indicate a stronger signal from the brain, but this is never interpreted on its own. FSH is always considered alongside other information, particularly AMH and ultrasound findings; it is the pattern between results that matters most, rather than any single number.

Radical honesty: A single high FSH result does not define anything. Stress, illness and timing can shift levels. Patterns matter more than moments.

If AMH is about how many eggs may be left, and FSH reflects how hard the body is working to recruit them, the next hormone helps your clinician understand whether ovulation is being triggered as expected.

Luteinising hormone (LH)

LH triggers ovulation and usually works in balance with FSH. When LH is significantly higher than FSH early in the menstrual cycle, it can suggest a pattern sometimes seen in PMOS (*see* pp. 30–31) or irregular ovulation. This may prompt clinicians to look a little more closely at how ovulation is being regulated.

Alongside LH, another hormone commonly measured early in the cycle is oestradiol.

Oestradiol

Oestradiol helps the uterine lining grow and supports egg development. It is often tested early in the menstrual cycle alongside FSH, because higher oestradiol levels can temporarily make FSH appear lower than it actually is.

On day two to three of the cycle, oestradiol is typically below 200pmol per litre. Higher levels at this point can make FSH results harder to interpret. An unexpected oestradiol reading is not a catastrophe. It is another piece of information that helps clinicians understand how your menstrual cycle is unfolding.

While oestradiol plays its role before ovulation, the next hormone is measured after ovulation to help confirm that ovulation has taken place.

Progesterone

Progesterone plays an important role in maintaining the lining of the uterus in preparation for possible implantation. A progesterone level above around 25–30nmol per litre measured in the mid-luteal phase (*see* p. 18) usually confirms ovulation. Lower levels may suggest that ovulation did not occur, that ovulation was weaker or that the timing of the blood test did not quite align with your progesterone peak.

Radical honesty: A low progesterone level is one of the most treatable findings in fertility care. Many people respond well to medication that supports ovulation or helps strengthen the luteal phase (the time between ovulation and your next period).

Once ovulation has been assessed, clinicians often investigate hormones that can interfere with the communication between the brain and ovaries, even when cycles appear relatively regular.

Prolactin

Prolactin is best known for its role in supporting milk production after birth. When prolactin levels are raised outside pregnancy, they can interfere with ovulation. Stress, poor sleep and some medications can raise prolactin, which is why a mildly elevated result is fairly common.

Prolactin levels are usually considered within the expected range when they are below 500mIU per litre. Mild elevations are often temporary and linked to everyday factors such as stress or medication use. Most raised prolactin levels are treatable, and bringing prolactin back into range can help support more regular ovulation.

At this point in testing, many clinics also check the thyroid. This is not because the thyroid sits within the reproductive system, but because it plays an important role in menstrual cycle regularity, ovulation and early pregnancy.

Testosterone

Although testosterone is often thought of as a male hormone, it is also produced by women and plays an important role in overall health and reproductive function. Low testosterone levels can sometimes be associated with reduced fertility, and emerging evidence suggests that testosterone supplementation may improve fertility outcomes in some women. As with all hormone testing, results should be interpreted in the context of an individual's wider clinical picture.

Thyroid function

Your thyroid is a small gland in your neck that has an enormous influence on hormones, energy levels, metabolism and menstrual cycles. Checking thyroid function is a simple way of making sure this foundation is steady before or during fertility treatment.

Thyroid testing usually includes a small group of related hormones. While the names can feel technical, each one is responsible for a slightly different aspect of thyroid function.

Thyroid-stimulating hormone (TSH)

TSH is the hormone your brain uses to guide the thyroid; it works a little like a thermostat. If the thyroid is underactive, the brain produces more TSH to encourage it to work harder. If the thyroid is overactive, the brain produces less TSH because the gland is already producing more hormone than needed.

This matters for fertility because even mild thyroid underactivity can interfere with ovulation, lengthen menstrual cycles, increase pregnancy loss risk and make early pregnancy harder to sustain. This is why fertility clinics often pay close attention to thyroid function.

Many fertility specialists aim for a TSH between around 1.0 and 2.5mIU per litre when supporting couples who are trying to conceive or undergoing treatment. The general population reference range is wider, often around 0.5–4.5mIU per litre. This means you may be told your thyroid is normal for general health, even when the level is not ideal for fertility.

Radical honesty: It can feel confusing to hear that your thyroid is 'normal' in one setting and 'suboptimal' in another. This reflects different goals. Fertility and early pregnancy often require tighter hormonal balance than day-to-day life does.

Free T4

Free T4 is one of the main hormones produced by the thyroid. It shows how much thyroid hormone is circulating and available for your cells to use. A normal or high normal free T4 alongside a raised TSH can suggest the thyroid is under strain. A low free T4 with a normal or high TSH can indicate underactive thyroid function that may benefit from treatment.

Free T3

Free T3 is the active form of thyroid hormone: the version your cells actually use. It is not always tested, but doing so can be helpful if symptoms continue despite normal TSH and free T4 levels, or if fertility treatment is not progressing as expected.

Thyroid antibodies

Thyroid antibodies include thyroid peroxidase (TPO) antibodies and thyroglobulin antibodies. They look for autoimmune thyroid conditions such as Hashimoto's thyroiditis, which is common and can go undetected for many years.

This matters for fertility because thyroid antibodies can affect ovarian function, implantation, early pregnancy development, pregnancy loss risk and unexplained infertility. Even when TSH levels are normal, positive thyroid antibodies may mean the thyroid needs closer support during fertility treatment or early pregnancy.

Alongside the hormones that regulate ovulation and the menstrual cycle, some clinics also look at a small group of hormones known as androgens.

DHEAS and testosterone

DHEAS (dehydroepiandrosterone sulphate) and testosterone are produced by the adrenal glands and the ovaries. They play a role in energy levels, hormone balance and the early stages of follicle development. These androgens sit slightly outside the core reproductive hormones, but they can still influence how the ovaries respond and how eggs develop.

Tests for these hormones are most often requested when ovarian reserve appears low, or when the ovaries are not responding as expected during treatment. In some people, very low levels of DHEAS or testosterone may be linked to poorer egg development or a reduced response to stimulation during IVF.

Reference ranges vary widely depending on age, sex and the laboratory used. As a broad guide:

- DHEAS levels for women often fall between 1 and 9 micromol per litre.
- Total testosterone levels are often below 2 nanomoles per litre.
- Free testosterone may also be measured to give a clearer picture (although the normal range can vary between laboratories depending on how it is calculated).

Rather than focusing on precise cut-offs, clinicians usually look at where your levels sit within the expected range for your age and how they fit with the rest of your results.

How this can guide treatment

Understanding androgen levels can help your team decide whether a supplement might be useful. This is sometimes recommended for people with low ovarian reserve to support egg development, but it is not appropriate for everyone and is not helpful when levels are already normal or high.

If used, the dose and timing need to be precise and should always be guided by a fertility specialist who understands your full hormone picture. Taking it without supervision can disrupt hormone balance rather than support it.

Radical honesty: DHEAS is a powerful hormone. More is not better.

At this stage in testing, once the main reproductive hormones have been reviewed, clinics often widen the focus a little. This is about checking the underlying foundations that support hormone balance, implantation and early pregnancy.

Other blood tests that support fertility care

These tests are not about egg number or ovulation directly. Instead, they look at the wider physical environment in which conception and pregnancy need to take place. Small imbalances here can quietly influence how the body copes with treatment and early pregnancy.

Vitamin D

Vitamin D plays a role in hormone balance, immune function and implantation. Low levels are extremely common in the UK, particularly during the winter months, and many people are unaware their levels are low until they are tested.

- Levels above 50nmol per litre are usually considered sufficient.
- Levels between 30 and 50nmol per litre are often described as insufficient.
- Levels below 30nmol per litre are typically considered deficient.

Clinics often aim for levels towards the higher end of the normal range when trying to conceive.

Full blood count

Alongside vitamin D, clinics usually check a full blood count. This provides a broad overview of how your body is functioning day to day and whether it has the resources it needs to support conception and pregnancy.

A full blood count looks at your red blood cells, white blood cells and platelets. It can highlight things like anaemia, infection or inflammation, which may affect energy levels, recovery and how well your body copes with pregnancy.

Typical values vary slightly between laboratories, but in general:

- Normal haemoglobin for women is around 120–160g per litre.
- Low levels of haemoglobin or small red blood cells can suggest iron deficiency.
- Raised levels of white blood cells may point to infection or inflammation.

Doctors are less interested in a single number and more interested in both the overall pattern and whether anything stands out that needs support.

Ferritin, B12 and folate

Because fatigue, low mood and poor recovery are so common during fertility treatment, clinics often look more closely at key nutrients that support energy and blood health. Ferritin reflects your iron stores rather than your circulating iron, while B12 and folate are essential for red blood cell production and early fetal development.

- Ferritin above 30 micrograms per litre is usually acceptable, though many fertility specialists aim for 50–100 micrograms per litre.
- B12 typically falls between 200 and 900ng per litre.
- Folate above 7nmol per litre is usually considered adequate.

If levels of any of these are low, they are usually straightforward to correct with supplementation. Addressing them early can make a noticeable difference to how people feel physically during treatment.

HbA1c and glucose

Some clinics also assess how your body handles blood sugar, particularly if your menstrual cycles are irregular, ovulation is inconsistent or PMOS (*see* pp. 30–31) is part of the picture. HbA1c gives an overview of average blood sugar levels over the past two to three months. Fasting glucose looks at how your body manages sugar in the moment.

- HbA1c below 42mmol per mol is considered normal.
- HbA1c between 42 and 47 suggests prediabetes.
- HbA1c above 48 indicates diabetes.
- A normal fasting glucose is usually below 5.5mmol per litre.

Radical honesty: Being told you have raised glucose or insulin resistance can feel worrying. For many people, though, this is one of the most modifiable findings. With the right support, menstrual cycles often become more regular and treatment response can improve.

Once these general health foundations have been checked, clinics usually move on to screening that helps protect both your health and the health of a future pregnancy.

Screening for infections

As fertility testing moves forward, clinics routinely screen for a small group of infections. This is a standard and preventative part of care, designed to protect your health, support implantation and reduce risks during treatment and pregnancy. Many of the infections screened for are extremely common and often cause no symptoms at all.

You may notice that some of these screening tests are repeated if you are freezing eggs, sperm or embryos, or if treatment is delayed. This is because clinics also have to meet strict laboratory safety regulations when storing reproductive cells, which are often kept in shared storage tanks. Screening allows samples to be handled and stored safely, and a positive result simply means additional precautions are taken. It does not prevent treatment or freezing.

With that context in mind, clinics usually begin infection screening with a small set of blood tests known as serology.

Serology

Serology refers to blood tests that check for certain viral infections, most commonly HIV, hepatitis B, hepatitis C and, sometimes, syphilis.

The results are usually reported as 'reactive' or 'non-reactive'. A reactive result does not mean treatment cannot go ahead. It means there will be further discussion, planning and support to ensure care is safe for you, your partner and a future baby.

Rubella immunity

Rubella screening checks whether you are protected against rubella, a viral infection that can cause harm if contracted in early pregnancy.

Rubella immunoglobulin G (IgG) above the laboratory threshold (often around 10–15IU per millilitre) indicates immunity. If immunity is not present, vaccination may be advised before trying to conceive.

This is a precautionary step and one that many people can take without issue.

Chlamydia

Chlamydia is one of the most common STIs in the UK. Most people who carry it have no symptoms and are unaware it is present.

If left untreated, chlamydia can lead to inflammation or scarring within the reproductive tract. In women, this can affect the fallopian tubes (*see* p. 40) or lead to PID (*see* pp. 41–42). In men, it can affect sperm health. It can also be passed to a baby during birth.

Testing is usually carried out via a urine sample or vaginal swab.

Gonorrhoea

Gonorrhoea is another common infection that can be present without symptoms. If untreated, it can cause PID (*see* pp. 41–42), tubal damage (*see* p. 40), reduced sperm quality and neonatal infection.

Testing is usually carried out through a urine sample or swab, depending on the clinic.

Ureaplasma and mycoplasma

These are less well-known bacteria that can live in the reproductive tract without causing symptoms. Many people carry them without ever knowing.

In some people, these bacteria have been linked to subtle inflammation, reduced sperm quality and early pregnancy complications. Testing is usually performed via a vaginal swab or semen sample.

Treatment and reassurance

The reassuring news is that most infections identified through fertility screening can be treated with a short course of antibiotics: often around five days, depending on the medication used. Where appropriate, partners are treated at the same time to prevent reinfection.

Although infection screening can feel confronting or uncomfortable emotionally, it is a routine part of good fertility care. It is about protection, not judgement.

Once infection screening is complete, and if fertility difficulties remain unexplained, clinics may then suggest looking at genetics to better understand whether inherited factors could be playing a role.

Genetic screening

Genetic screening looks for inherited conditions you may carry without ever knowing, such as sickle cell disease, thalassaemia or other recessive conditions. Testing is usually offered based on ethnic background, family history or clinic policy, and is carried out via a simple blood test or cheek swab.

What these tests look for

Most conditions included in genetic screening panels follow a recessive inheritance pattern. This means you can carry a genetic change without having the condition yourself. It only becomes relevant if both partners carry a change in the same gene.

Genetic screening does not use numerical values. The results usually fall into one of two categories:

- Not a carrier
- Carrier of a specific gene variant

If you are identified as a carrier, your partner may be offered screening too. This is not because anything is wrong. It is simply about understanding the full picture so that informed choices can be made if needed.

> **Radical honesty: Genetic screening can naturally bring up 'what if' questions. What matters most is remembering that genetic information offers clarity and choice. It does not remove your chance of becoming a parent, nor does it decide your future. For many people, it simply provides reassurance.**

For a small number of people, genetic screening may lead clinicians to suggest a more detailed look at the chromosomes themselves.

Chromosomal karyotype

A chromosomal karyotype is a blood test that looks at the number, size and structure of your chromosomes. You can think of it as a photograph of your genetic filing cabinet. It shows whether each pair of chromosomes is present, intact and arranged in the expected way.

Why it is performed in fertility care

A chromosomal karyotype is usually suggested when there are signs that it may help explain repeated or unexplained difficulties, such as:

- Recurrent pregnancy loss.
- Repeated implantation failure.
- Very low sperm count.
- A family history of certain genetic conditions.
- Unexplained infertility despite normal test results.

Sometimes, one partner carries a chromosomal rearrangement, such as a balanced translocation (*see* p. 49). In this situation, all of the genetic material is present but arranged differently. This often has no impact on the person's own health but can make conception or early embryo development more challenging.

What the results might show

- Normal karyotype: The chromosomes appear structurally and numerically typical.
- Balanced translocation: All genetic material is present but arranged differently, which can affect embryo development.
- Sex chromosome variations: Examples include Klinefelter syndrome (*see* p. 93), where an extra X chromosome may influence sperm production.

What it may mean emotionally

Discovering a chromosomal variation can stir many feelings. Shock, confusion, grief or even guilt are common first reactions, even though these patterns are inherited and entirely outside your control.

Please hold on to this:

You did not cause this.

You could not have prevented it.

And there are still clear and achievable paths forward.

Options such as IVF with genetic testing, or the use of donor eggs or sperm (*see* pp. 186–90) if that ever feels right for you, can lead to healthy pregnancies and healthy children.

A chromosomal karyotype already represents a deeper level of genetic investigation. Very occasionally, and particularly when answers remain unclear, clinics may suggest more advanced genetic testing to look for explanations that standard tests cannot show. This is not common, and for most people, the investigations outlined above provide sufficient clarity to move forwards.

From here, it can be helpful to understand how access to fertility testing works in the UK.

Where to go for fertility testing: NHS and private pathways

In the UK, some fertility tests are available through the NHS, while others are offered only when certain criteria are met. This can feel confusing, particularly when you are ready for clarity and want to understand what is happening as quickly as possible.

NHS fertility care usually follows a stepwise approach. Most people begin with basic assessments such as hormone blood tests, an ultrasound scan and a semen analysis. Further investigations are added only if you have been trying for a certain length of time, if you have experienced recurrent pregnancy loss or if early results suggest that something needs closer attention. More detailed tests, such as genetic screening or advanced diagnostics, often take place in private clinics.

It is completely understandable to feel frustrated if NHS pathways move more slowly than you would like. Many people describe a strong sense of urgency at this stage of their fertility journey, and the structure of NHS care can feel out of step with that urgency. This is not because your GP or specialist does not care. NHS services must follow national guidance, local criteria and population-level priorities, which means they cannot always offer every test at the moment you feel ready for it.

A FEW THINGS THAT ARE HELPFUL TO KNOW

- The NHS will usually start with the basics: hormone tests, an ultrasound scan and a semen analysis.
- More specific tests, such as AMH, tubal assessments or genetic screening, may be offered only if there is a clear medical reason or if you meet certain time-based criteria.
- Advanced diagnostics such as chromosomal karyotyping (*see* p. 76) are rarely offered unless earlier investigations point strongly in that direction.
- Private clinics can often offer a wider range of tests sooner, as they are not bound by the same thresholds or waiting times.

Understanding this structure can help explain why a particular test may not be offered when you first ask for it. It does not mean the test is unimportant. It reflects the pathway you are expected to move through.

Hold in mind:

You are still allowed to advocate for yourself.

You are allowed to ask why something is or is not being offered.

You are allowed to request clarification or a second opinion.

And you are allowed to seek private testing if you feel it would give you clarity or help you move forwards more confidently.

Before we move on, it may help to pause and look at some of the questions people commonly have at this stage.

Common questions about fertility tests

What is the most important fertility test?
There is no single most important test. Fertility reflects a combination of egg quality, sperm health, ovulation, hormonal balance and the health of the uterus and fallopian tubes. The clearest understanding comes from looking at how these factors interact.

Why are some of my results marked as 'abnormal' when my doctor says they are fine?
Laboratory reference ranges apply to the general population. Fertility clinics use narrower ranges that relate specifically to ovulation, implantation and early pregnancy. This is why interpretation matters more than the number itself.

Do my hormone levels change every month?
Yes. Hormones fluctuate naturally. Stress, illness, sleep and the timing of the blood test can all affect results. This is why clinicians often repeat tests or look at patterns over time.

Will a low AMH or high FSH mean I cannot get pregnant?
No. These results describe ovarian response, not your future. Many people with low AMH or high FSH conceive naturally or with treatment, and many people with normal results still need support.

Why does my partner need testing if my results already look abnormal?
Fertility challenges can involve one partner or both partners at the same time. Even when one set of results already explains part of the picture, it is still important to assess sperm health because

male factors contribute to around half of fertility difficulties overall. Understanding both sides together helps create the clearest picture, avoids missing additional issues and supports the most appropriate treatment decisions.

If I change my lifestyle, will my hormone levels improve?
Some hormone levels, such as thyroid function, insulin regulation or vitamin D, may respond to lifestyle changes. Others, such as AMH, do not usually increase in a meaningful way. Lifestyle supports overall health but cannot reverse ovarian ageing.

Should I track everything?
Only if it helps you. For some people, tracking brings reassurance. For others, it increases pressure. If tracking heightens your anxiety, it is reasonable to step back and let your medical team guide the process.

Will testing lead straight to treatment?
Not usually. Testing gathers information. With that information, you can decide calmly what your next steps are, whether that means continuing to try naturally, addressing a treatable issue or considering treatment.

What if I feel overwhelmed by my results?
This is very common. Results often carry emotional weight. Take your time. Ask for explanations more than once if needed. Share how you are feeling with someone you trust. These results are information, not judgement.

Final reflections

It is very common to try to make sense of your entire fertility story from a single result. This is also one of the quickest ways to feel overwhelmed or misled, because fertility does not work like that. Almost no test in this chapter is meaningful on its own:

- AMH speaks to quantity, not quality.
- FSH is influenced by timing and stress.
- Progesterone only makes sense in relation to ovulation.
- An ultrasound is a snapshot, not a prediction.
- A semen analysis can change within weeks.

The real value of testing comes from seeing how the pieces fit together. A good clinician looks at your age, medical history, hormone patterns, ultrasound findings and menstrual cycle history, your partner's results and, sometimes, genetics. It is the relationship between these factors that guides decision-making.

It can also help to remember that most results reflect function, not fate. They describe how your body is working right now, not what will or will not happen in the future. Many findings are treatable, and others can be worked around with the right support.

You now have an overview of what fertility tests look for, how they are used and why they matter. These tests are tools that help build a clearer picture of what is happening in your reproductive system. As you continue, the most useful thing you can do is stay curious and keep asking for explanations that make sense to you.

If we may, we would invite you to pause here, just for a moment.

Fertility testing can bring up a lot: relief, worry, confusion and hope, sometimes all at once. If you feel unsettled, that does not mean you are doing anything wrong. It means this matters to you. Take your time, and be gentle with yourself. This is a lot to hold, and we want you to know that we understand how overwhelming it can feel. While results can be hard to face, having clearer information is often the first step in making sense of what is happening and taking back a little more control.

As we move forward, it is important to remember that fertility is never just about one body. In the next chapter, we turn our attention to the male factor's role in fertility.

4

Male fertility: we see you

If you are reading this as a man, we want to begin with a very simple message: you are not a side character in this process. You are not just the person who waits outside the scan room or provides a sample when asked. You are part of this story in full. Your biology matters. Your experience matters. Your voice matters.

For a long time, fertility has been spoken about as if it belongs mostly to the female body. Leaflets, websites and support groups often focus on menstrual cycles, hormones, follicles and eggs. None of that is wrong, but it means something important can be missed. You may recognise this. Men often find themselves quietly pushed to the edges of their own story.

This is why it can feel so shocking when a semen analysis shows something unexpected. It may also stir up a particular kind of guilt. If your partner is having blood tests, scans or medications, you might look at those procedures and feel as if she is carrying the physical burden while your results have added another layer of difficulty. You may find yourself worrying that she is going through all of this because of something in your body, even if neither of you could have known or prevented it.

These thoughts are understandable. They can feel heavy, and they can create worry about whether any of this reflects on you personally. It does not. It reflects biology. And biology can be understood and worked with.

You deserve clarity, care and space. You deserve a chapter that speaks directly to you. So, let us explore male fertility together.

Understanding male fertility

Most men, like most women, have never been taught how their reproductive system works. That is not your fault. In the UK, education usually focuses on preventing pregnancy rather than explaining how it actually happens. As a result, many men reach adulthood with little sense of what sperm are, how they develop or what influences their quality.

In this chapter, we will explore the most common reasons sperm may be absent or reduced, including structural issues, ejaculatory factors, hormonal influences and genetic causes. Understanding these different pathways can help make sense of where difficulties arise and why specific tests or treatments may be recommended.

How sperm are produced

Sperm production is a finely balanced process that depends on several parts of the body working together. The brain sends signals through hormones that tell the testicles to produce sperm. The testicular tissue needs a good blood supply so that oxygen and nutrients can reach the cells in the testicles responsible for making sperm. The temperature of the scrotum needs to remain slightly cooler than the rest of the body for sperm cells to grow properly. Even the environment around the developing sperm matters, because it influences how well the cells mature and whether they are damaged along the way.

This process does not happen quickly. It takes around three months for sperm to develop from the earliest stage to the point where they can fertilise an egg.

Semen analysis

Because sperm takes around three months to develop in your body, a semen analysis reflects what has been happening over that period of time, rather than just on the day the sample is given. This means that the sperm sample you give on any one day is a reflection of the past few months of your life. How you slept, what you ate, how stressed you were, whether you were unwell and even the amount of heat around your testicles all play a part in shaping the result. It also means that sperm quality is not 'fixed'. Instead, it can change. And that is an important part of the story.

Understanding what you can do to prepare for the test and what the test looks for can help you make sense of the results in a calmer and more grounded way. We will explore this now.

Preparing for a semen analysis

There are a few small steps you can take to prepare for a semen analysis that will help make the test as accurate as possible:

- Try not to ejaculate for two to five days beforehand.
- Avoid heavy alcohol use in the few days leading up to the test.
- Avoid saunas, hot baths or anything that overheats the testicles for 72 hours before the sample.
- If you are unwell or have had a fever recently, let the clinic know, as this may affect the results.

These simple steps will help ensure that the test reflects your typical sperm quality rather than a temporary change. Once you have a sample that represents your body as it is, it becomes much easier to understand the numbers in front of you.

Understanding a semen analysis

A semen analysis is usually the first step in understanding male fertility. The test itself is straightforward, but the terminology can feel unfamiliar. Words like concentration, motility, morphology and vitality may look technical, yet each one describes a specific part of how sperm form and function. We will look at these more closely now. Remember: none of these results say anything about your character. They simply reflect what was happening in your body over the last three months.

Volume

This is the amount of fluid in the sample. Most men fall somewhere above about 1.4ml. A lower volume can happen if you were dehydrated or anxious, at the time of producing or if you had ejaculated recently. Sometimes, a lower volume of fluid points to a blockage in the ducts that transport semen, but most of the time it is a normal variation.

Concentration

Often called the 'sperm count', this measures how many sperm are present in each millilitre of semen. A concentration above around 16 million per millilitre sits within the typical range used by UK clinics. Concentration can vary from sample to sample and is influenced by hormones, heat exposure, illness, past injury or genetics. A lower sperm count can arise for many reasons. Hormones from the brain may be fluctuating. A varicocele (*see* p. 90) may be increasing heat around the testicle. You may have had a fever or viral illness in the weeks before the test. Some medications can temporarily reduce the sperm count. In other cases, the ducts that carry sperm may be blocked or, more rarely, may have been absent from birth (*see* p. 90). Sperm count is one of the parameters most affected by stress, poor sleep and heat exposure.

Motility

Motility describes how well the sperm move. UK reference ranges suggest that total motility above about 42 per cent is typical, with at least 30 per cent moving progressively forwards. Motility is sensitive to lifestyle factors such as smoking, vaping, alcohol, heat and stress, and also to medical conditions like varicocele (*see* p. 90). Sometimes, motility is lower simply because the sperm have been affected by illness, dehydration or long gaps between ejaculations.

Morphology

Morphology refers to the shape and structure of sperm. In semen analysis, sperm are assessed with regard to what proportion have a typical shape. A figure above 4 per cent normal forms is considered typical; this can feel surprising, because it means the majority of sperm appear irregular. Morphology varies widely and, on its own, does not strongly predict natural conception. Most samples contain a high proportion of unusual shapes, even in men who conceive naturally. Slight variations in head or tail shape often do not cause issues. Severe abnormalities can point to genetic or developmental causes, but in many men, morphology alone does not predict fertility.

Vitality

Vitality measures how many sperm in the sample are alive. This helps clarify whether reduced motility is due to sperm not moving well or simply not surviving.

White blood cells

A raised number of white cells may indicate inflammation or infection. This is usually temporary, treatable and not necessarily linked to long-term fertility issues.

INTERPRETING YOUR RESULTS

The WHO reference ranges (standards published by the WHO that laboratories use to measure and interpret semen analysis →

results) used in UK clinics describe what is typical across the general population. They are not pass or fail results. If one or more parameter sits outside the range, it simply means there is something to explore. It does not mean you have caused the issue or that things cannot improve.

A semen analysis is a starting point, not a verdict. What matters is not one number on one day but what those numbers mean in the context of your overall health, your partner's fertility and the steps you take together.

Acute and reversible causes of suboptimal results

It is worth remembering that sperm parameters fluctuate. Sperm parameters are sensitive to what has been happening in your body over the past few months. Short-term changes, even those you might not connect with fertility, can have a noticeable effect on a semen analysis. This is why repeating a semen analysis (*see* pp. 86–87) is often recommended before drawing firm conclusions.

Fever

A high temperature, even for a short period, can temporarily reduce sperm count and motility. This may not show up until several weeks after the illness, because sperm take time to mature.

Recent illness

Viral infections, flu, COVID-19 or any illness that places strain on the body can affect the developing sperm. Recovery from most of these changes happens gradually over the following months.

Intense exercise

Periods of very intense training, particularly endurance sports or heavy weight-lifting, can temporarily reduce sperm count or testosterone. When training returns to a balanced level, sperm quality often improves.

Alcohol bingeing

Heavy drinking over a short period can cause a temporary drop in sperm motility and increase DNA damage. Regular moderate drinking is less likely to have the same effect.

Recent smoking or vaping increase

If your smoking or vaping increased in the weeks before the test, it may have affected sperm movement and DNA quality. Smoking and vaping can negatively affect sperm count, movement and genetic health, which may impact both natural conception and fertility treatment outcomes. Stopping smoking and vaping is strongly recommended for anyone trying to conceive, as reducing or stopping can make a meaningful difference to fertility and long-term health over time.

Stress

Stress does not cause infertility, but it can influence hormone regulation, sleep, appetite and recovery, which all feed into sperm production. A particularly difficult season can show up in the semen analysis results.

Heat exposure

Prolonged exposure to heat around the testicles, such as saunas, hot baths or heated car seats, can temporarily reduce sperm count and motility.

Medications

Some medications, especially testosterone supplements, anabolic steroids, certain psychiatric medications and previous chemotherapy, can reduce sperm production. The effect depends on the medication and how long it is used.

Radical honesty: These factors are common, temporary and often reversible. If any of them have been part of your recent life, repeating the semen analysis after a few months may give a clearer picture of your long-term fertility.

When to repeat a semen analysis

Because semen parameters naturally fluctuate, a single test rarely gives the full picture. Repeating the analysis helps you and your clinical team understand whether the first result reflects your usual sperm health or a temporary change. It may be helpful to repeat the test if:

- You had a fever or illness in the previous three months.
- You had a long gap between ejaculations before the test.
- You were under significant stress or sleeping poorly.

- You were unwell on the day of the test.
- You had recently increased alcohol use, smoking or vaping.
- The sample was difficult to collect.
- You have made lifestyle changes, and you want to see their effect.

Repeating the test is not about checking whether you have done 'better'. It is simply a way of understanding your biology more clearly and making decisions based on the most accurate information.

When you can see which factors might be temporary, it becomes easier to understand what you can influence more directly. One of the more hopeful parts of male fertility is that sperm respond to the environment they develop in. Small, steady shifts in how you care for your body can lead to meaningful changes over time.

Hormonal testing for men

Hormones are central to sperm production. They act as signals that tell the testicles when to begin producing sperm and how much to produce. A simple set of blood tests can provide useful information about these signals, especially if your semen analysis shows changes in concentration, motility or sperm survival.

When a semen analysis shows changes, blood tests may be used to look more closely at the hormones that control sperm production. The hormones below are the most commonly checked, as they help explain how signals from the brain and testes are working together.

Follicle-stimulating hormone (FSH)

FSH is one of the main messengers from the brain to the testicles. A higher-than-expected FSH level can mean that the brain is working harder than usual to stimulate sperm production. This can happen when the testicular tissue is under strain. A lower FSH level can suggest the opposite: that the signalling from the brain is quieter than it needs to be.

Luteinising hormone (LH)

LH works alongside FSH and helps stimulate testosterone production. LH and testosterone are closely linked, so if one is outside the expected range, the other is often checked to understand the full picture.

Testosterone

Testosterone supports many aspects of male health, including sperm development, sex drive and energy levels. Most men with fertility difficulties will still have testosterone levels in the typical range, but if the level is low, it can affect the speed or quality of sperm production. A testosterone level that is too high, especially as a result of supplement or anabolic steroid use, can also reduce sperm production.

Sex hormone binding globulin (SHBG)

SHBG affects how much free, active testosterone is available in the body. A high SHBG level may make testosterone appear lower than it truly is in terms of availability. This test helps clarify the overall hormonal picture.

Prolactin

Prolactin is another hormone produced in the brain. When it is higher than expected, it can interfere with testosterone production and sperm development. Mild increases are common and often linked to stress, sleep disruption or certain medications.

Thyroid function

Thyroid hormones support many processes in the body, including metabolism and energy regulation. When thyroid function is significantly underactive or overactive, it can indirectly affect fertility. Testing is usually carried out if symptoms or other blood results suggest a thyroid imbalance.

Understanding these hormones can help you and your clinical team see whether the signals between the brain and the testicles are working smoothly. It also helps identify when a hormonal imbalance might be contributing to the semen analysis results.

Structural factors

Alongside hormones, it is also important to consider the physical structures within the testicles and scrotum that are involved in transporting and producing sperm. These structures develop early in life and often cause no symptoms at all, which means many men are unaware that anything may be different. A simple examination or scan can bring useful clarity.

Sperm production and transport depend on a network of small tubes, blood vessels and tissues within the scrotum. When any part of this system is affected, the semen analysis may change. These structural causes are common and often straightforward to understand once they are explained.

Varicocele

A varicocele is a cluster of enlarged veins in the scrotum. These veins can raise the temperature around the testicle and increase oxidative stress, both of which can affect sperm count, motility and DNA quality. Some men feel a dragging or heavy sensation, while others notice nothing at all. Varicocele is one of the most common structural findings in male fertility care.

Obstruction of the vas deferens

Sperm are produced in the testicles but must travel through the vas deferens, a small duct that carries them towards the urethra. If this duct becomes blocked due to infection, inflammation or injury, sperm may not appear in the sample even though they are being produced.

Congenital absence of the vas deferens

Some men are born without one or both vas deferens. This absence can be associated with changes in the *CFTR* gene (*see* p. 93), which is also linked to cystic fibrosis. Men with this finding usually feel well and produce sperm normally, but because the ducts are absent, the sperm cannot leave the testicle. Surgical sperm retrieval is often possible if needed.

Previous testicular torsion

Testicular torsion occurs when the testicle twists, cutting off its blood supply. It is usually very painful and requires urgent treatment. Even when corrected quickly, torsion can affect sperm production later in life, particularly on the side where the twist occurred.

Undescended testes

If one or both testicles did not descend into the scrotum during childhood, or if this was corrected later, sperm production may be reduced. The testicle develops best at the cooler temperature of the scrotum, so being inside the abdomen early in life can have long-term effects.

Trauma

A significant injury to the testicles, even many years ago, can influence sperm production. Many men do not immediately link past injuries with current fertility results until the subject is explored in an assessment.

These structural findings form just one piece of the picture. Another part involves what appears in the sperm sample itself, as previously discussed (*see* pp. 83–85).

When no sperm appear in the ejaculate

Sometimes, a semen analysis shows no sperm at all. This result is called azoospermia. It can feel alarming at first, especially if you have no symptoms, but azoospermia has various causes (as discussed below) and does not always mean that sperm are not being produced.

Obstructive azoospermia

In this situation, sperm are being made but cannot leave the testicle. This can happen when:

- The vas deferens is blocked.
- The vas deferens is absent from birth.
- There has been a previous infection or inflammation.
- Retrograde ejaculation is occurring (*see* p. 92).
- Previous surgery or trauma affected the ducts.

Men with obstructive azoospermia often feel well and have normal hormone levels and testicular size. In many cases, sperm retrieval via a minor procedure is possible.

Non-obstructive azoospermia

Here, the difficulty lies within the testicular tissue itself. Sperm may be produced in very low numbers or not at all. Causes include:

- Genetic conditions, such as Y chromosome microdeletions (*see* p. 93) or Klinefelter syndrome (*see* p. 93).
- Long-standing testicular damage.
- Severe hormonal disruption.

Even in cases of non-obstructive azoospermia, sperm retrieval may still be possible in the hands of a specialist, because small areas of active sperm production can sometimes be found.

Retrograde ejaculation

During orgasm, the semen travels backwards into the bladder instead of forwards through the urethra. This can be caused by:

- Nerve changes resulting from diabetes.
- Previous prostate surgery.
- Certain medications.
- Spinal or pelvic nerve injury.

Men with retrograde ejaculation often notice cloudy urine (which contains sperm) after sex. Treatment may involve new medication, adjusting existing medication or collecting sperm from the urine for use in treatment.

Anejaculation

Anejaculation is when ejaculation does not occur at all despite orgasm or sexual arousal. Causes include nerve conditions, certain medications, psychological factors or long-standing patterns of delayed ejaculation. Support from a urologist or sexual health specialist is often helpful.

Why understanding the underlying cause matters

These conditions can sound alarming when first explained, but they provide clear information about where the difficulty is arising. They also open the door to specific treatments and options, including sperm retrieval, medication changes or assisted reproductive techniques such as intracytoplasmic sperm injection (ICSI; *see* pp. 184–85).

Understanding these structural and ejaculatory factors can help you see that difficulties with sperm production or transport have many possible explanations. Alongside these, genetic influences play a role in how sperm develop. These findings are usually discovered through simple blood tests and can offer important clarity about what is happening in your body.

Genetic causes

Some fertility difficulties originate from the way in which certain genes influence reproductive development. These findings are not common, and many men with these diagnoses have lived their whole lives in good health with no symptoms. When identified, they help your clinical team understand why sperm production looks the way it does and how best to support you in the next steps.

Y chromosome microdeletions

The Y chromosome carries genes that are important for sperm production. In some men, very small sections of this chromosome are missing. These are called microdeletions. Depending on which section is affected, sperm production may be reduced or, in some cases, absent. A simple blood test can identify this.

Klinefelter syndrome

Klinefelter syndrome occurs when a man is born with an extra X chromosome (so their chromosomes are XXY rather than the typical male XY). Many men with this condition are not diagnosed until adulthood, and most live healthy, active lives. Klinefelter syndrome can reduce testosterone levels and affect sperm production. Hormonal support or surgical sperm retrieval may still be possible in some cases.

CFTR gene changes

The *CFTR* gene is linked to cystic fibrosis. Some men who carry certain *CFTR* changes may be born without the vas deferens, the ducts that carry sperm out of the testicles. These men usually produce sperm normally, but the sperm cannot reach the ejaculate. Sperm retrieval is often possible, and IVF with ICSI (*see* pp. 184–85) is commonly used.

Genetic findings can feel unsettling at first, simply because the language is unfamiliar. What matters most is that they provide clear information about where the difficulty is arising. They also help your team guide you towards the most effective and appropriate options.

It is also worth remembering that not all changes in sperm quality point to long-standing or complex causes. Some are temporary, reversible and linked to everyday events in your life (*see* pp. 86–87). These factors can influence a semen analysis for weeks or months, and they often improve on their own once the body has recovered.

When to see your GP, fertility clinic or urologist

You do not need to navigate this alone. Different professionals can help at different stages, and understanding their roles can make the next steps feel calmer and more manageable. Let's look at who you can turn to for help.

Your GP

Your GP is usually the first point of contact. They can arrange an initial semen analysis and basic blood tests, and they can give you an overview of lifestyle factors that may be relevant. If a result sits outside the typical range, most GPs will repeat the test after a few weeks or refer you to a fertility clinic for more specialised assessment.

Your fertility clinic

Fertility clinics can provide a deeper level of testing. They may repeat the semen analysis, assess DNA fragmentation, check your hormone levels in more detail and explore whether structural factors such as varicocele may be contributing. They will also look at your results alongside your partner's to understand the whole picture. Clinics can guide you through treatment options and help you decide what feels right.

A urologist or andrologist

If your results are significantly outside the expected range, or if there are structural, hormonal or genetic questions that need specialist input, a referral to a urologist or andrologist (a specialist in male reproduction) can be helpful. These specialists can examine the testicles and ducts, request targeted scans or genetic tests and advise on whether treatments such as varicocele repair, hormone therapy or surgical sperm retrieval might be appropriate.

WHEN TO CONSIDER SEEKING SPECIALIST SUPPORT

It may be time to speak with a specialist if any of the following apply:

- Sperm count is persistently very low, or sperm is absent.
- A significant structural cause is suspected.
- Your hormone levels are unusual.
- You have had a previous testicular surgery or injury.
- Conception has not happened after a year of regular sex.
- You simply want clearer information and a more detailed plan.

Reaching out for specialist support is not an escalation. It is a step towards understanding your body in a clear, grounded way and deciding what path feels right for you.

Once you understand your results and have spoken with the right professionals, the next step is often to explore what treatment options might support you. This can feel like a big moment, especially if you have never imagined you might need medical help to conceive. The aim of the next section is not to overwhelm you but to give you a clear sense of what each option involves and why it might be recommended.

Treatment options

Fertility treatment is not one single path. The right option depends on the cause of the difficulty, your partner's fertility and your hopes as a couple. A number of options are available, which are explored in chapter 8. Each of these options may be supported by either medical or surgical interventions, which we discuss below.

Medications that may support sperm production

There are times when medication can gently nudge the hormonal system into a better rhythm. These treatments are not used for everyone, but they can be helpful when blood tests show a hormonal imbalance or when sperm production needs additional support. They work by improving the signals between the brain and the testicles or by supporting testosterone in a way that enhances, rather than suppresses, sperm development.

Clomifene citrate

This medication encourages the pituitary gland to release more FSH and LH, the hormones that stimulate testosterone production and sperm development. It is often offered in situations where the hormonal signals are quieter than they need to be. Though it is a simple tablet, it can have a meaningful effect on both testosterone levels and sperm count.

Letrozole

Originally developed for breast cancer treatment, letrozole can help redirect the balance of hormones in a way that increases natural testosterone levels. For some men, this shift improves both sperm count and motility. Its use in male fertility has grown as we have begun to understand just how responsive the hormonal system can be.

Gonadotrophins

These injectable hormones provide direct stimulation for the testicles to produce sperm. They are particularly effective when the body is not producing enough FSH and LH on its own. Treatment requires commitment and regular monitoring, but for some men the improvement in sperm production is significant.

These medications may be available through NHS services when male factor infertility is clearly demonstrated, although access varies across the UK. If you believe hormonal support may help, it is worth discussing this openly with your GP or fertility specialist. Clear information and a referral to a urologist or andrologist can help you understand whether medical treatment is an appropriate next step.

There are also times when a structural issue can be treated surgically. Understanding these options can help you see where further support may lie.

Surgical treatments that may improve fertility

Some fertility difficulties arise from issues that cannot be addressed through lifestyle changes or medication alone. In these situations, specific surgical procedures may help improve sperm quality or allow sperm to be retrieved for treatment. These interventions sound technical, but when explained clearly, they offer practical routes forward.

Varicocele repair

A varicocele is a cluster of enlarged veins that can warm the testicle and disrupt sperm production (*see* p. 90). Repairing these veins can lower the temperature, reduce oxidative stress and improve sperm count and motility. For some men, this procedure leads to meaningful improvements in natural conception or treatment success.

Vasectomy reversal

If you have previously had a vasectomy and would now like to pursue pregnancy, a surgical reversal may reconnect the vas deferens and allow sperm to reappear in the ejaculate. This option depends on how long ago the vasectomy was performed and the condition of the ducts; however, for many men, it offers a realistic way forwards.

Surgical sperm retrieval techniques

When sperm do not appear in the ejaculate, retrieving them directly from the epididymis or testicle can be an option. Procedures such as microsurgical epididymal sperm aspiration (MESA), testicular sperm extraction (TESE) or micro-TESE allow surgeons to locate areas of active sperm production. If sperm are found, they can be used for ICSI (*see* pp. 184–85) or frozen for future treatment cycles. These techniques depend on the underlying cause and require detailed specialist assessment, but they offer hope when ejaculation is not possible or when sperm production is very low.

Again, these procedures are available in some NHS centres, although access varies according to local funding and expertise. Many men choose to explore private options, where waiting times may be shorter and techniques such as micro-TESE are more widely available. Whatever route you take, make sure you understand how the procedure will be performed and what the plan is for storing or using any sperm that are retrieved.

After looking at the different medical and surgical options, it can be helpful to step back for a moment and remember that behind every decision is a real person trying to understand what these possibilities mean in day-to-day life. Treatments and techniques are important, but they make sense only when they sit within someone's actual experience. To bring this into focus, below is the story of one man who found himself navigating these questions in his own way.

CASE STUDY: JAMES – MALE FACTOR FERTILITY

James was 34 when he and his partner attended a fertility clinic after more than a year of trying to conceive. He had always assumed things would work naturally, so when the clinic suggested a semen analysis, he expected it to be routine.

The results surprised him. His sperm concentration was lower than expected, and the motility was reduced. His partner's tests looked reassuring, which made him worry that the weight of their difficulty now rested on him. He felt confused, embarrassed and unsure how to speak about it.

Further assessment helped make sense of the findings. His hormone tests showed that his brain was working harder than usual to support sperm production, and a small varicocele was warming the testicle more than it should. None of this had caused symptoms. He had simply never known these issues were there.

With clearer information, James made some small changes. He adjusted his training, reduced his alcohol intake, focused on sleep and had the varicocele reviewed. Three months later, his semen analysis looked different. Not perfect, but improved enough for the clinic to suggest moving ahead with ICSI.

What changed things for James was not only the treatment. It was the shift from feeling at fault to understanding the biology behind his results. Once he knew what was happening and why, he no longer felt alone or ashamed. He felt informed, involved and part of the process again.

James's experience is one example of how complex this journey can feel. It can also highlight how much this process lives within a relationship. With that in mind, it may help to think about how you and your partner move through this together.

Working together as a couple

Fertility difficulties rarely affect one person alone, even when the medical findings point towards male factor causes. You and your partner may be experiencing the results of male factor testing differently, at different speeds and with different emotions. That is normal. It can also be a place where you strengthen your connection.

Many men worry about saying the wrong thing or feel unsure how to speak openly about their results. You do not need perfect language. What helps most is honesty in small, manageable steps. You might say something like, 'I am still taking this in, but I want us to go through it together', or 'I care about this, and sometimes I find it hard to express what I feel.' These simple statements can create more closeness than you expect.

Your partner may also be carrying worries of her own, and she may be trying to protect you at the same time. Opening a conversation, even gently, can give both of you room to share what this experience is bringing up. You can take turns, pause when you need to and come back to the conversation later. It does not need to be resolved in one sitting.

It can also help to decide together how you want to handle appointments, results and decisions. Some couples prefer to read information separately and talk when they are ready. Others find it helpful to sit together, read the results at the same time and make notes for the next appointment. There is no right or wrong approach. What matters is that your approach feels supportive to both of you.

If the two of you find communication difficult at times, it does not mean your relationship is weak. It means you are human and facing something that touches deep hopes and vulnerabilities. Speaking with a counsellor at your clinic or a therapist outside the clinic can help create a safe space for both of you to think, talk and breathe.

You do not have to navigate this alone, and you do not have to carry all of it silently. Working together does not remove the difficulty, but it often makes it more bearable.

After taking in so much information, it can be helpful to slow the pace for a moment and return to the centre of what this chapter is really about. Behind every number, every test and every option is a person trying to make sense of a situation they did not expect. You may still be processing your own results or wondering what they mean for your future. Wherever you find yourself, be kind to yourself and give yourself the time you need to let everything settle. And if you need support, it is okay to ask for it. As you begin thinking about next steps, one of the most important decisions ahead may be choosing where you receive your care, and whether that environment feels safe, supportive and right for both of you.

5

Choosing your clinic:
how to find a place where you feel safe, supported and understood

Before we talk in any detail about treatment plans or medical decisions, we need to pause at a crucial practical point: choosing where you will have treatment. If you are at this stage, it usually means you have already had the initial tests and conversations, and you have begun to shift from wondering to deciding. This part can feel both exciting and daunting, and, as we often say, both feelings can exist at the same time.

We believe that choosing where you will have treatment is not only a practical decision; it is an emotional one. It asks you to place hope and trust, and often a significant investment of time, energy and money, into a team of people you do not yet know. It is a decision that touches your body, your future family and one of the most vulnerable chapters in your life. You may already have a clinic in mind, or you may have been offered a referral and be wondering whether it feels right for you.

You are not already meant to know how to make this choice. Most people reach this point feeling unsure, even if they have already done the tests and the waiting. It is common to worry about choosing the wrong place, not knowing the right questions to ask or not fully understanding the differences between clinics or between NHS and private care. You may also wonder whether it is acceptable to expect emotional support alongside medical expertise.

All of these feelings and questions are normal. This chapter is here to help you feel more grounded as you decide what matters most to you, and to guide you through the practical considerations in a clear, manageable way.

Why choosing the right clinic matters

A clinic is not just a building or a service. It becomes the backdrop to some of the most vulnerable moments of your life. It is where you may receive news that breaks your heart or news that makes you hopeful again. It is where you will ask questions about your body, your hormones, your embryos and your future. It is where you may experience uncertainty, fear, courage and relief all in the same day.

Choosing the right clinic is not about finding perfection. It is about finding somewhere that feels safe, that has the necessary medical expertise and that is supportive enough and human enough for you. The place you choose can shape all of the following:

- How seen and understood you feel.
- How clearly your treatment is explained.
- How respected you feel in decisions about your body.
- How emotionally supported you are.
- How connected you feel to your partner or support system.
- How realistic your expectations become.
- How you navigate stress, hope and disappointment.

The clinic you choose should ultimately intertwine your emotional and physical experience. When you choose a clinic that meets both of these elements, the journey becomes steadier. Not easier necessarily, but steadier.

> **Radical honesty: A clinic with excellent success rates but poor communication or limited emotional support may still leave you feeling frightened and alone. A clinic with warmth but limited transparency can leave you confused or mistrustful. You deserve a clinic that fulfils all of your needs.**

In essence, you are looking for warmth and clarity. Kindness and competence. Humanity and science. So, let's have a think together about how to go about finding this.

Do you choose the clinic or the treatment first?

People tend to worry that they should already know what treatment they need before choosing a clinic. This is not true. You are not expected to know the medical route first. In almost every case, the order is as follows:

1. You choose the clinic.
2. The clinic helps you understand which treatment is right for you.

You should not need to self-diagnose, nor do you need to arrive prepared with a plan. Your only responsibility at the beginning is to find a place that feels safe enough for you to start to understand what choices are available to you.

Your choices within the UK system

In the UK, you can choose between NHS-funded care and private treatment. Trying to make this decision can feel like standing at a crossroads with no signposts. Both paths have strengths and limitations. Both can offer excellent medical care. Both can also feel confusing or frustrating depending on your circumstances.

Let's make this as clear and gentle as possible.

NHS care

The NHS offers fertility treatment based on local eligibility criteria, which means your access depends on the region where you live (also known as the 'postcode lottery'; *see* p. 103). These criteria often include:

- Age.
- Body mass index (BMI).
- Existing children.
- Length of time trying.
- Whether you are using donor sperm as a same-sex couple or a single parent.
- Medical history.

Waiting times can be long. You may wait months for an initial appointment and longer before treatment begins. When you are ready to move forwards and are feeling the pressure of time, these waits can feel unbearable.

However, NHS clinics also provide:

- Experienced medical teams.
- Highly regulated laboratory standards.
- Clear eligibility pathways.
- Good safety oversight.

If you qualify and can tolerate the wait, NHS care can be an excellent starting point.

NICE GUIDANCE ON FERTILITY TREATMENT

In the UK, national guidance on fertility treatment is produced by the National Institute for Health and Care Excellence (NICE). NICE provides recommendations on who should be offered fertility treatment and how many IVF cycles should be funded by the NHS.

The guidance recommends:

- Up to three full cycles of IVF for women under 40 who have been trying to conceive for two years (or after 12 cycles of artificial insemination).
- One full cycle of IVF for women aged 40 to 42, provided certain clinical criteria are met.
- A full cycle includes the transfer of any embryos created during that treatment cycle.

However, NICE guidance is not mandatory. Local Integrated Care Boards decide how fertility treatment is funded in their area, which is why access varies across the country.

For practical steps on how to check the criteria where you live, *see* 'How to Check Your Local Criteria' later in this chapter.

The postcode lottery

You may have heard the phrase 'postcode lottery' when people talk about fertility treatment. It describes the simple but painful reality that, as we mentioned above, access to NHS-funded fertility care varies depending on where you live. This is not because your situation is less important or your medical need is different; it is simply because different geographical areas offer different levels of support.

The reality is that if you are accessing NHS-funded care, your choice of clinic may be limited. In some parts of the country, you may be offered a small selection of clinics, but in many areas, there is only one option. This is because NHS fertility care is organised and funded by your local Integrated Care Board (ICB). Every region of England has its own ICB, and each one decides who is eligible for treatment and with which fertility clinics they hold contracts. Your referral usually goes to the clinic your ICB works with rather than to the clinic you might have chosen for yourself.

Once you know this, it becomes clearer why some people receive several NHS-funded treatment cycles (rounds of fertility treatment), while others receive none. The differences can be stark. One area may follow the national guidance in full.

Another may offer limited treatment. Another may not fund treatment at all. Two people with almost identical medical histories can face completely different pathways, purely because their homes fall on different sides of a geographical boundary. This is incredibly hard to digest if you live in a less favourable postcode.

Many people assume NHS fertility care is the same everywhere, and discovering that it is not can bring disappointment, frustration and a sense of being left out of something you expected to rely on. It can feel restrictive, especially if the clinic you are allocated to does not feel like the right emotional or interpersonal fit. You may find yourself comparing it to private clinics you have seen online or worrying that you will not receive the kind of support you have hoped for.

Understanding the postcode lottery is not about asking you to accept it as fair, because it is not. Instead, it is about helping you understand why your options may be narrower, or why waiting times or funding may look different from what you have heard elsewhere. We hope that having that clarity will help you plan your next steps.

Radical honesty: You may need to ask directly to find out what is possible. Some options are not offered automatically, even when they are available in your area.

How to check your local criteria

If you are unsure what your area offers, there are two simple ways to find out. The first is to search online for your local ICB alongside the words 'fertility policy' or 'assisted conception policy'. Most ICBs publish their criteria openly. The second is to ask your GP or the clinic handling your initial investigations. They can tell you which clinic(s) your area uses, what treatments are funded and whether there are age, BMI or relationship criteria you need to know about.

Private care

Private clinics offer:

- Shorter waiting times.
- Flexibility with appointment scheduling.
- A wider range of treatments.
- More comprehensive communication.
- Greater choice of clinics and clinicians.

However, private care also comes with costs that can be significant, and sometimes unexpectedly so. Medications in particular can vary dramatically in price depending on pharmacy and protocol.

> **Radical honesty: Paying privately can give you more choice and faster access to treatment, but it does not automatically guarantee better communication, emotional support or a more personalised experience. A clinic can have excellent success rates and still not feel like the right fit for you. You deserve to feel informed, respected and cared for, regardless of how your treatment is funded.**

If you are paying privately, you can choose any licensed clinic in the UK. You can research, visit, compare and change if something does not feel right.

Both pathways have strengths and challenges. NHS care is funded and often provides excellent medical care, but waiting times can be long and criteria vary by postcode (*see* p. 103). Private care offers faster access and more flexibility, but it comes with significant cost.

> **Radical honesty: In the UK, access to treatment varies by region, and cost often shapes the options available to people. Private clinics can offer shorter waiting times and more flexibility, but they are not affordable for everyone.**

Combining NHS and private care

If the NHS-funded support in your area is limited, it does not mean you have no choices. Some people choose to continue NHS investigations while exploring private treatment. Others mix the two pathways. For some people, it is possible to use both NHS and private care at different points, although this depends entirely on the policies in your area. In some regions, the NHS will continue to offer certain investigations or blood tests even if you plan to fund treatment privately. In others, moving into private care means the NHS part of your pathway closes. Your GP or clinic can explain what is possible where you live.

When it is available, mixing pathways might look like beginning your investigations through the NHS and choosing private treatment if waiting times feel too long. It might mean being monitored through the NHS while treatment itself happens privately, although this is not offered everywhere. Some people also return to NHS services for early pregnancy care, which is usually straightforward no matter where they received treatment.

There is no single formula here. What is possible depends on your postcode and the arrangements in place locally. If you are considering combining NHS and private pathways, ask your GP or clinic what support they can offer so you have a clear picture of what is realistic for you.

You are not powerless. You are entitled to ask questions, to request clarity and to let the team know what helps you feel supported. And if the environment truly does not feel right for you, it is possible to fund part or all of your care privately, either at the same clinic or at a different one. It is also worth saying that many NHS clinics provide excellent care, even when the system itself limits your freedom of choice at the beginning.

Financial costs of private fertility care

The financial side of private treatment can be uncomfortable to think about, especially when you are already managing so many emotions. But it is an important part of the picture, and understanding it early often brings more clarity and less shock later on.

Private fertility care is made up of several different costs, some of which are predictable and some of which depend on how your treatment cycle unfolds. The main areas to be aware of are outlined below.

The consultation

This is your first appointment with the doctor. Fees vary between clinics, but many people pay between £200 and £400. This usually includes a medical review and recommended next steps.

Investigations

These include blood tests, scans, semen analysis and any additional assessments your clinician feels are necessary. Some tests are inexpensive, while others can cost several hundred pounds. These tests often need repeating over time. Ask for a clear estimation of what your treatment will involve.

Treatment fees

This is the core cost of IVF or ICSI. The fee usually, but not always, covers monitoring scans, blood tests, egg collection, fertilisation in the laboratory and embryo transfer. Prices vary widely between clinics and regions. It is not unusual for a single IVF treatment cycle to cost several thousand pounds.

Medication

Medication is often one of the biggest expenses. Costs vary depending on your protocol, your dose and the length of treatment. Some people spend hundreds, others thousands. Clinics will usually give you a prescription so you can compare pharmacy prices if you wish.

> **Radical honesty: It is completely acceptable to shop around for your medication. Some clinics offer medication at a fair price, while in other cases you may find it more cheaply through a pharmacy. You are not being difficult or disloyal by comparing costs. You are simply looking after your resources at a time when every decision carries weight.**

Laboratory fees

Some procedures in the laboratory carry additional fees. These can include embryo freezing, time-lapse imaging, assisted hatching or genetic testing. The cost depends on the technique and how many embryos you have. It is important to consider these upfront.

Storage fees

If you freeze your eggs or embryos, most clinics charge yearly storage fees. These vary, but they are an ongoing cost you need to plan for.

Early pregnancy care

Some clinics include follow-up scans and early pregnancy monitoring in the treatment fee. Others charge separately for these services.

The important thing here is not memorising the numbers, it is knowing that private treatment is made up of layers of cost, not one single fee. A good clinic will explain this clearly from the start, showing you what is included and what is not, so you can plan realistically rather than being surprised midway through.

You also have every right to ask whether there are payment plans, packages for multiple treatment cycles or refund schemes, and whether they are appropriate for someone with your circumstances. These options can sometimes help, but they are not suitable for everyone, and you should never feel pressured into choosing them. This is why transparency matters.

TRANSPARENT COST CHECKLIST

- Consultation fees
- Investigation costs
- Medication costs (which can be significant)
- Treatment fees
- Pregnancy monitoring fees, including scans
- What is not included
- Payment options
- Add-ons (*see* chapter 9)

Money is rarely spoken about openly in fertility clinics, yet it quietly shapes decisions every day. It can feel confronting to realise that your treatment choices sometimes depend on finances rather than medical need. This is a hard reality of a system where many people must self-fund.

You do not need to have everything figured out in advance. But gaining clarity around costs can reduce anxiety and help you make decisions rooted in care rather than panic.

A supportive place to start can be to ask your clinic for a detailed breakdown of fees. Many headline prices do not include medication, monitoring scans, embryo storage or early pregnancy appointments. An itemised quote helps you understand the full picture so that no cost takes you by surprise. You may want to consider:

- Treatment fees, including stimulation, egg collection, fertilisation and transfer.

- Medication costs, which can vary by hundreds of pounds between pharmacies.
- The price of additional scans, tests or add-ons if recommended (the latter often causes confusion and is worth investigating early; *see* chapter 9).
- Storage fees for embryos or eggs.
- Time away from work for appointments, procedures and recovery.
- Travel costs and childcare, if relevant.

Radical honesty: Many people fund treatment through credit cards, loans or payment plans. Others use savings, remortgage or receive help from family. Some pause treatment to recover financially. These choices reflect how deeply people want a child and how costly this path can become.

Our aim here is not to tell you how to spend your money. It is to encourage you to make decisions with clarity rather than urgency. Financial decisions made in panic can bring regret later, whereas decisions made slowly and consciously often feel kinder.

INSURANCE COVERAGE

Private medical insurance rarely includes fertility treatment, sadly. Some policies cover initial investigations like blood tests or semen analysis, but IVF and IUI are usually excluded unless the employer provides a highly specialised plan. For most people, this means treatment is either self-funded or accessed through the NHS, as we have discussed.

When you know the practical boundaries of what is available to you, the next questions become more personal: what kind of clinic would feel right for you, and what matters most in the space where you will be cared for? Let's explore that.

What makes a good clinic

A good clinic is not defined by a stylish Instagram presence, impressive branding or the most expensive price list. A good clinic is one where you feel safe. One where your voice matters, and where you understand what is happening to you rather than feeling lost in jargon or pressure.

Here are some of the qualities that we feel truly matter. Perhaps have a think about what stands out to you and keep notes, if that helps.

Respect for your autonomy

You should feel that your decisions belong to you. This means that your clinic should be guiding you, not directing you. Supporting you, not steering you. A clinic that respects your autonomy will:

- Explain all appropriate options, not just the most expensive ones.
- Check your understanding.
- Invite your questions.
- Give you time to think.
- Welcome a second opinion.
- Never shame you for choosing differently.

It should feel like a respectful collaboration.

> **Radical honesty: Your clinical team may be experts in fertility treatment, but you are the expert in your body and your life. Good care holds both forms of expertise with equal respect.**

Clear, honest, open communication

Fertility medicine carries uncertainty, so honesty and transparency are vital. You should feel that the information you receive is evidence-based, realistic and kind. A clinic should:

- Explain success rates in a way you understand.
- Be transparent about risks and limitations.
- Avoid making inflated promises.
- Speak plainly, without jargon.
- Provide written information you can read later.
- Offer clear timelines and expectations.

Our hope is that you never leave an appointment bewildered or more confused than when you arrived.

> **Radical honesty: A clinic that is proud of its outcomes will be open to explaining them.**

Emotional and psychological support

Fertility treatment can be emotionally demanding, and clinics vary in how they support this aspect of care. It is important to choose a clinic that reflects your expectations of what emotional wellbeing should look like during the process. Emotional support might look like:

- Access to fertility-focused counsellors.
- Staff who speak gently and without dismissal.
- Clinicians who acknowledge fear and uncertainty.
- Space to talk about loss, disappointment or anxiety.
- Your partner being included in conversations.
- Reception and nursing teams who recognise the human being in front of them.

What does emotional support look like for you?

Everyone's needs here are different. Some people feel steadier when they have close guidance at each stage. Others prefer a quieter, more hands-off approach where information is given clearly but without frequent check-ins. You may already know what helps you feel supported, or you may still be working that out. Either is completely fine.

Radical honesty: Whatever your style of coping, one thing holds true for almost everyone: kindness matters. It should be present in every interaction and should never be something you have to compromise on.

It can be helpful to begin thinking about the kind of emotional environment that feels most grounding for you. Much of that comes down to the people caring for you.

A team that feels right

This is something you cannot measure on paper, and it can be subjective. Be mindful of things like:

- The tone.
- The warmth.
- The willingness to listen.

- The space they give you to breathe.
- The way they respond when you ask a difficult question.

Your experience of the doctors and other staff

The people involved in your care play an important role in how you experience treatment. Skill and experience matter, but so does the way in which you are spoken to and the feeling you get from the team around you. A clinician might be very knowledgeable yet leave you feeling rushed. Another might take more time to explain things in a way that helps you feel steadier. Both aspects are part of good care.

In some clinics, especially within the NHS, you may meet different members of the team across appointments. This is common and does not mean your care is disjointed. What helps is having a clear sense of who is guiding your overall plan and feeling that the information about your care is shared consistently between staff.

Radical honesty: If the relationship with a member of your clinical team does not feel right for you, it is acceptable to ask to see someone else. This is about your comfort and your care.

A GENTLE CHECKLIST FOR YOURSELF

When you interact with a clinic, you might quietly ask yourself the following questions:

- Do I feel listened to?
- Do I understand what is being explained?
- Do I feel calmer or clearer afterwards?
- Do I feel like a person rather than an appointment slot?
- Do I feel that my emotional needs matter here?

If you answer no to several of these, it may be a sign to keep looking.

Perhaps this is a good moment to pause and notice how all of this is landing for you. There is a lot to take in, and it is completely natural to feel a mixture of clarity, relief, worry and even information overload. Whatever has come up for you is valid.

When you are ready, we can move into the practical side of things.

How to choose a clinic: practical steps

Understanding what makes a good clinic is one part of the process. We believe that the next part is knowing how to move through the practical steps in a way that feels like you are in control rather than overwhelmed.

Here is a practical way to approach choosing your clinic.

Step one: start with the HFEA

(Human Fertilisation and Embryology Authority)

In the UK, every fertility clinic must be licensed and regulated by the HFEA. Their website and data allow you to compare clinics in a standardised way, without marketing language or selective data. On the HFEA website, you will find:

- Success rates.
- Inspection reports.
- Patient ratings.
- Clear explanations of treatment options.
- Evidence ratings for add-ons (*see* chapter 9).

You do not need to analyse the numbers like an expert, unless you want to. You are simply looking for consistency, safety and transparency. If one clinic has repeated warnings or concerns raised in inspections, this is useful information. If another clinic shows strong patient ratings year after year, that also tells you something important about the human experience of care.

Perhaps think of the HFEA as your first filter. It helps narrow the landscape so you can focus your energy on choices that are truly viable for you.

Step two: build a shortlist

We suggest that once you have a sense of the landscape, you can begin creating a shortlist of clinics that may suit your situation. When people reach this stage, they often feel pressure to find the single perfect clinic. But as we say, the goal is not perfection; instead, the goal is to find a few clinics that seem safe, accessible and appropriate for you.

You might consider:

- Location and travel time.
- Whether you are eligible for NHS-funded care at that clinic.
- Which treatments they offer.
- Whether the clinic has a satellite location closer to you.
- Waiting times for initial appointments.
- Patient reviews (with the awareness that reviews tend to represent extreme experiences).

Try to approach this step gently, as you are simply gathering possibilities.

Step three: book an initial consultation

The initial consultation is a point where many people want to feel prepared, and this book is here to help with that. Even so, you are not expected to know everything or to speak in medical terms. The consultation is a guided conversation, and it should feel spacious enough for you to ask questions, pause, reflect and notice how you feel about the place.

In the consultation, notice how the clinician speaks to you. Notice the pace. Notice whether the explanations feel clear. Notice whether the questions they ask feel tailored to you or repeated by rote.

This consultation is your opportunity to get a sense of the clinic's tone. Some clinics have a calm, thoughtful pace. Others feel hurried or transactional. Some clinicians lean into empathy. Others focus heavily on data. None of this is wrong in itself, but it helps you understand whether the style fits your own individual emotional needs.

In the next section (*see* pp. 116–18), we have suggested some questions you may wish to ask at your initial consultation.

Step four: notice how you feel afterwards

When you leave the clinic, pause before diving into logistics or numbers. Ask yourself quietly:

- How do I feel in my body?
- Did I feel respected?
- Did the conversation leave me grounded or overwhelmed?
- Did the clinician seem to understand my specific situation?
- Did I feel rushed or pressured?

- Did I feel able to ask for clarity?
- Did I leave with a sense of partnership or a sense of distance?

We believe that these internal cues can be some of the most reliable information you will ever gather. You may not identify the feeling immediately, but you will recognise a subtle shift. This could look like a small expansion in your chest if you feel safe, or a quiet tightening if you did not. Take a moment to observe your responses.

CASE STUDY: ELLA AND MIA – THE INITIAL CONSULTATION THAT DID NOT SIT WELL

Ella and Mia, a same-sex couple, chose a well-known clinic with a strong reputation for supporting LGBTQ+ families. They arrived at their first consultation feeling prepared and hopeful.

During the appointment, the clinician directed almost all of their questions and explanations towards Ella, who planned to carry the pregnancy. Mia was present, engaged and ready to contribute, yet the focus remained almost entirely on one partner. The clinician spoke about results, next steps and treatment options without involving Mia in a meaningful way.

Nothing explicit was said, and nothing overtly inappropriate occurred, but the imbalance was noticeable. Mia left with a quiet sense of unease, unsure whether the clinic would fully include her in decisions that affected them both. Ella also sensed the dynamic and felt concerned about what this might mean for the rest of their treatment experience.

After the appointment, they took time to reflect. Although the clinic was highly regarded and specialised in working with couples like them, the consultation had raised questions about communication, inclusivity and whether they would feel equally supported throughout treatment.

They decided to look elsewhere and booked another consultation. At the next clinic, both partners were included naturally in the conversation, their questions were welcomed and the consultation felt balanced and respectful. This contrast confirmed their decision to switch.

For them, noticing that something did not sit well early on helped them choose a clinic that aligned better with their expectations and offered the sense of partnership they needed.

Questions to ask your clinic at the initial consultation

Before we move on, we want to give you something practical and grounding. Many people worry they might forget what to ask or feel overwhelmed in the moment. When you are sitting in a consultation, it is easy to lose track of what matters to you, especially if the conversation becomes heavy with statistics or medical language. The pace can also feel quicker than you expected.

To help you feel steady and organised, we have put together a list of questions that you can use as a guide. These questions are there to support you and to help the clinician understand what you need. They create space for a more individual conversation rather than one based only on numbers or test results.

Feel free to think of the questions below as options, not as an essential list. They are tools for clarity. You can choose the ones that feel relevant, save others for later and set aside anything that does not apply to you. If there are questions we have not included, make a note of them and add your own.

Questions about treatment:

- Based on what you know so far, what treatments might be suitable for me and why?
- Are there other options I should consider?
- What are the steps involved from the beginning to embryo transfer, and then what happens?
- How do you adjust treatment if things do not go as expected?
- How often will we review progress?
- What about add-ons?

Questions about success and outcomes:

- What are your success rates for someone my age or with my diagnosis?
- How do you calculate those rates?
- How many people like me reach embryo transfer?
- What are your pregnancy loss and live birth rates?
- How do your results compare to national averages?
- What happens next if the first treatment cycle does not work?

Questions about waiting times:

- What is the average wait for investigations?
- What is the average wait for starting treatment?
- What influences these timelines?
- What happens if I need to move more quickly?

Questions about costs:

- What is the full expected cost, including medications and pregnancy monitoring?
- What is not included in that quote?
- Do you offer payment options or plans for multiple treatment cycles?
- What are the costs of add-ons, and what evidence supports them?

Questions about communication and staff:

- Who will be my main contact person?
- Will I always see the same clinician, where possible?
- How do you deliver results?
- How quickly do you respond to messages?
- How are weekends and bank holidays covered?
- What should I do if I need urgent advice?

Questions about emotional support:

- What emotional support do you offer?
- How does counselling work here?
- How do you support donor conception decisions?
- Are there any peer or group supports I can access?
- How do you include partners if they want to be involved?

Questions about laboratories and technology:

- How do you keep laboratory standards high?
- Who are your embryologists, and will we meet them?
- What technologies do you use to assess embryos?

Questions about ethics and future decisions (if applicable):

- What are your policies on donation, surrogacy and storage?
- What happens to embryos if treatment is paused?
- How do you help with longer-term decisions?

Questions about aftercare:

- What support do you offer after a treatment cycle?
- Do you debrief after unsuccessful treatment cycles?
- How do you support early pregnancy?

And finally, one question that we firmly believe is worth asking:

- If I were your daughter, your sister or your friend, what would you recommend for me?

This question often reveals the clinic's heart more clearly than anything else. All of this information is here to support you. Now let's turn it into something you can use. All of this information is here to support you in making decisions that feel informed, practical and right for your circumstances. For some people, those decisions may also include exploring treatment outside the UK.

Considering treatment abroad?

For some people, treatment abroad becomes part of the conversation. This may be because waiting lists in the UK feel too long, because donor availability is limited, or because the laws around donation differ. In the UK, all donors are identity release, meaning a donor-conceived child can access identifying information about the donor at eighteen. In some other countries, anonymous donation is still permitted, which leads some patients to explore treatment elsewhere. Clinics abroad may also offer larger donor banks, different matching systems or shorter waiting times.

If you are considering this route, it is important to understand that each country has its own laws around donation, embryo storage and parentage. Practical considerations matter too. You may want to check whether consultations and documents are available in English, what exactly is included in the cost of treatment, and how follow-up care will work once you return to the UK. Travelling for treatment can bring additional emotional and logistical demands, so it can help to think carefully about what will feel manageable and supported.

In summary

As you reach the end of this chapter, we can probably all agree that choosing a fertility clinic is not just a practical step; it is a personal one. And it is one that asks you to think about what you need, what you value and what makes you feel steady in a process that can feel anything but.

In these pages, we have looked at what shapes this decision. We have talked about how a clinic makes you feel, how to understand success rates, how to recognise red flags, how to approach NHS and private care and how to think about cost and travel, as well as how emotional support fits into all of this. We have also touched on treatment abroad and the questions that can help anchor you in your appointments.

The purpose has never been to overwhelm you. It has been to give you a clearer sense of what matters for you. If there is one thing to hold on to, it is this: you are allowed to choose the clinic that feels right for your needs and your circumstances. The clinic where you feel listened to, respected and able to ask questions. The clinic that gives you a sense of safety, however fragile that feeling may be at the start.

This is your body and your journey. You deserve care that meets you with clarity and humanity.

When you are ready, we will take the next step together. We want to help you feel as prepared as you can, and that's what the whole next chapter is dedicated to.

6

Preparing for treatment:
a guide to caring for your body and mind

If you are preparing to begin fertility treatment, you may already be hearing a lot of advice about what you should or should not be doing: how to eat, how to move your body, how to manage stress, what supplements to take and how to think and feel. This advice will be coming from many directions at once: friends and family wanting to help, social media feeds full of confident claims, podcasts, books and even clinics themselves, each emphasising different priorities. While much of this is well intentioned, it can quickly become overwhelming and contradictory, and you may find it difficult to know what actually matters.

Most clinics will have their own bespoke guidance, and some will offer personalised advice. To cut through this, we want to give you a clear, evidence-based foundation to help you understand what genuinely makes a difference to your physical and emotional wellbeing, amid the noise and advice that surrounds fertility treatment.

Before we step into the practical details, it is helpful to pause and consider the landscape you are navigating. You have more influence than you may realise. While there is much in fertility that cannot be controlled, there are parts of this process that sit firmly within your reach. The choices you make in the months before treatment can support both your physical and your emotional health.

Radical honesty: Sperm take around 70–90 days to develop, and during this time they are sensitive to lifestyle choices such as nutrition, sleep and stress. For eggs, the supply is fixed from birth, but the follicle that will release an egg goes through a period of

preparation in the months before ovulation. This means the three-month window before fertility treatment can be a meaningful time to support both sides of the process.

This chapter is divided into two parts: the first focuses on how to support your body, and the second focuses on how to support your mind. Although they are presented separately, they are deeply connected. The body and mind shape each other continuously. Caring for your physical health without tending to your emotional world can leave you feeling unbalanced, while caring for your emotional wellbeing without supporting your body can create unnecessary strain. We believe that working with both offers a more integrated foundation.

What you will find in this chapter is not a prescription; you do not have to follow every suggestion, and you certainly do not have to get everything right. Think of this chapter as a guide rather than a rulebook for preparing your mind and body. Over many years of working in fertility, we have seen consistent patterns in what supports the body and calms the mind. These are the adaptations that tend to make a meaningful difference, and, at the time of writing, they align with the best available evidence.

Some of what we suggest may feel familiar, and some parts may feel new. All of it is offered with the intention of helping you create the strongest, kindest foundation possible as you move towards the next stage of your journey. Feel free to take what supports you and leave what does not. This is your path and your preparation, and you get to shape it in the way that feels most aligned with you.

But before we begin, we wish to explore one area that has transformed the fertility world in the past decade, with implications for both your physical and mental wellbeing: social media.

Social media and the impact of online fertility advice

In many ways, the impact of social media has been extraordinary. People who once carried their journey privately now find whole communities that understand them. Women document their injections, their bruises, their early scans, their heartbreak and their joy. Men speak openly about sperm health and male factor infertility. Couples tell stories that were once whispered only inside clinic rooms. The silence around fertility has softened, and that visibility has changed everything.

Shared stories have offered comfort, solidarity and courage. They have helped people feel less alone. They have challenged stigma. They have allowed people to say, 'This is happening to me too', without shame. That is powerful. And yet, visibility has also brought noise.

Alongside the support sits misinformation. Confident non-experts share bold medical advice. Algorithms favour emotional content rather than accurate content. A video can go viral even if it is scientifically incorrect. A success story can sound like a guaranteed route. Something with soft music and a hopeful message can seem credible when the science beneath it is uncertain.

Radical honesty: Not all online fertility advice is harmful, but not all of it is safe.

When someone is hurting or desperate for answers, quick fixes are tempting. It is human to want hope. It is human to try one more supplement, one more diet, one more protocol seen in a reel at 3 a.m. Hope makes us resourceful, but it can also make us vulnerable. And this is where grounded preparation matters.

What we want to gently offer is this. If you follow accounts that soothe, educate and help you feel held, keep them. If you follow accounts that leave you frightened, flooded or pressured to buy and self-diagnose, you can unfollow. Curate your online world in the same thoughtful way you curate your healthcare team. And if Instagram says one thing but your clinic says another, ask. Bring these questions into appointments. A good clinic will never fear curiosity. They will welcome it.

Social media makes this journey less lonely, and that is a gift. But your medical pathway is not shaped by popularity or followers. It is shaped by evidence, individual context and what is therapeutically right for you.

Part 1: caring for your body

This part of the chapter will help you consider how you eat, sleep, move and live as you approach treatment. These everyday choices might seem small, but during the three-month window of egg and sperm development, they can influence the environment in which hormones are regulated, eggs and sperm mature and medication eventually takes effect. You are not being asked to overhaul your entire life. You are being invited to make changes that are realistic and sustainable.

Although fertility involves many layers, the body sits at the centre of the process. Menstrual health, hormone balance, egg and sperm development, metabolic rhythms and underlying conditions all contribute. Your lifestyle can support these processes. Food, movement, rest, alcohol, nicotine, environmental exposures and certain medications all influence how your body functions. None of this is about blame or judgement; instead, we focus on areas where small decisions can help your body feel better supported.

Please remember that preparing well is not about striving for an ideal version of health. It is about working with the body you already have and giving it the conditions it needs to do its job as effectively as possible. Within that, we hope you can find a rhythm that feels manageable and kind.

Nutrition

Nutrition is not about extreme rules or cutting out everything you enjoy. It is about giving your body what it needs to support hormonal balance, reduce inflammation and create the best possible internal environment for treatment.

Food provides the raw materials your body needs for egg development, hormone production and healthy implantation. We support the idea that the three-month window before ovulation is especially important. As you have probably realised, nourishment does not guarantee success; however, it does support your physiology in meaningful ways.

Below are the key elements of nourishment that can support your body's natural processes in the months before a treatment cycle.

For women

Antioxidants

Found in colourful fruits, vegetables, herbs, nuts and seeds.

Women's eggs are sensitive to something called oxidative stress, which is essentially a build-up of tiny molecules that cause cell damage. Antioxidants help protect against this and support healthy maturation.

Healthy fats

Found in olive oil, avocado, oily fish, walnuts, chia seeds and flaxseeds.

Hormones are made from fat, so the quality of the fats you eat directly influences the balance of oestrogen and progesterone (*see* p. 222). Healthy fats support hormone production, reduce inflammation and improve blood flow to the ovaries and uterus.

Complex carbohydrates

Found in oats, quinoa, beans, lentils, brown rice and whole grains.

Your hormonal system relies on stable blood sugar for smooth communication. Complex carbohydrates help keep insulin steady, which in turn supports ovulation, energy and mood regulation.

Protein

Found in eggs, oily fish, tofu, Greek yoghurt, poultry, beans and pulses.

Both egg development and hormone production rely on a steady supply of amino acids. Protein provides these building blocks, supporting egg quality, tissue repair and recovery during treatment.

Hydration

Water plays a surprisingly important role in preparing the body for treatment. It supports blood flow to the reproductive organs, helps regulate temperature, maintains cervical mucus quality and allows hormones to circulate more efficiently.

Aim for steady hydration throughout the day. Adding lemon, mint or herbal teas can help if water becomes repetitive.

Alcohol, caffeine and treats

Alcohol raises inflammation and disrupts hormone regulation. Moderation is usually appropriate, but minimising intake in the three months before treatment gives your reproductive system a clearer, calmer baseline.

Caffeine affects cortisol and sleep, which can influence hormonal rhythms. Keeping it within a moderate range helps maintain balance without feeling restrictive (under 200mg a day is considered safe).

Occasional treats do not undermine fertility preparation, and reducing pressure around eating can support a healthier stress response.

Enjoying food is part of wellbeing!

An anti-inflammatory pattern of eating

The dietary approach that supports fertility most reliably is one that keeps inflammation low. Inflammation can interfere with hormone regulation and implantation. An anti-inflammatory approach reduces this strain and supports the entire reproductive system. This approach to eating involves:

- Eating plenty of vegetables, berries and colourful fruit.
- Eating oily fish two or three times a week.
- Using olive oil as the main fat.
- Opting for whole grains rather than refined ones.
- Eating beans, lentils, pulses, nuts and seeds.
- Reducing intake of ultra-processed foods.
- Lowering consumption of refined sugars.
- Choosing alcohol sparingly.
- Keeping caffeine intake moderate.

This kind of diet can feel restrictive, so let yourself decide what is truly realistic for you right now.

Gluten free or dairy free?

Some people notice improvements in inflammation, energy or digestive comfort when they reduce or remove gluten or dairy, especially if they have endometriosis (*see* pp. 36–39), autoimmune conditions (*see* pp. 52–53), unexplained infertility (*see* pp. 55–58), PMOS (*see* pp. 30–31) or a reduced ovarian reserve. The research is evolving, and these changes are not required for everyone. What matters is how *your* body responds. Many people tolerate dairy well. Others find that dairy contributes to bloating, skin flare-ups or a sense of heaviness, and reducing it feels supportive. Gluten-free and dairy-free options are widely available across the UK, including when eating out, which makes experimentation easier.

> **Radical honesty: Gluten-free or dairy-free eating is only helpful if your physiology responds well to it.**

For men

As you know, sperm are constantly regenerating, and they complete an entire development cycle roughly every 70–90 days. This means that the choices made in the three months before treatment can meaningfully influence sperm quality.

How food supports male fertility

Sperm health depends on cellular integrity, energy production, hormonal balance and protection from oxidative stress. Nutrition provides the raw materials for these processes, and even small shifts can help.

Antioxidants

Sperm are particularly sensitive to oxidative stress, which can damage their DNA and reduce motility. The antioxidants found in berries, citrus fruits, leafy greens, tomatoes, peppers, herbs, nuts and seeds help protect sperm cells during their development.

Healthy fats

Olive oil, avocado, oily fish, walnuts, chia seeds and flaxseeds support hormone production, especially testosterone. They also improve the fluidity of the sperm membrane, which is essential for movement and fertilisation.

Protein

Steady sources of protein from eggs, oily fish, poultry, yoghurt, beans and lentils help support cellular repair and contribute to healthier sperm structure and function.

Complex carbohydrates

Whole grains, beans, lentils, vegetables and fruit help stabilise blood sugar levels. Stable insulin levels support hormonal regulation, which is important for sperm production.

Micronutrients

Sperm quality is responsive to zinc, selenium, vitamin C, vitamin E and folate, which support DNA integrity, motility and overall sperm volume. These micronutrients can be obtained through a varied diet, without the need for extremes.

Alcohol, caffeine and treats

Alcohol has a measurable impact on sperm health. Regular drinking can reduce sperm count, slow motility and affect shape, and these effects are often reversible when alcohol is reduced or paused. For many men, cutting alcohol intake significantly in the three months before treatment offers the most benefit.

Radical honesty: Sperm quality is one of the most changeable parts of fertility. For many men, even modest improvements in diet, alcohol habits and lifestyle can lead to meaningful improvements in semen analysis results. If you are unsure where to start, or if you have had a previous low result, speak to your doctor or a fertility dietitian who can tailor their advice to your needs.

Weight and metabolic health

Weight is a sensitive topic, and it can easily become loaded with judgement or shame. Yet it belongs in this section because metabolic health influences fertility in quiet but meaningful ways. Being significantly underweight or overweight can affect ovulation, hormone regulation, egg development and the way the body responds to fertility medication. In men, metabolic health can also influence sperm production, hormone balance and overall sperm quality. These effects are physiological, not moral.

You can think of metabolic health as the body's ability to regulate energy smoothly. When this system is steady, hormones communicate more reliably and menstrual cycles tend to be more predictable. When it is strained, menstrual cycles can become irregular, inflammation increases and treatment may require higher doses of medication. Supportive habits include all of the following:

- Eating balanced meals with protein, fibre and healthy fats.
- Keeping blood sugar steady through regular meals.
- Moving your body most days in ways that feel comfortable.
- Prioritising deep, consistent sleep.
- Reducing stress (which drives cortisol-related weight changes).

None of these require restriction or intensity. They are gentle, sustainable shifts that help your metabolism work more efficiently.

Radical honesty: You are supporting the internal rhythms that will guide your treatment. Even small improvements in metabolic balance can make a meaningful difference.

As you can see, the nutritional foundations for egg and sperm health are clear, practical and highly responsive to change. These are the areas where gentle, consistent choices can genuinely make a difference over the three-month development window.

Now that you have a sense of how food and weight support both egg and sperm development, we can turn to the next area people often ask about: supplements. This part of the journey can very quickly feel confusing, and it affects both partners.

Let's have a look at this in a little more detail.

Supplements and fertility

If you have ever typed 'best supplements for fertility' into Google, you will know how quickly the noise becomes overwhelming: long lists of 'must-haves', influencer bundles, medical language that is hard to decipher and products promising guaranteed success. It can leave you feeling as though you are missing something important or that you have fallen behind before you have even begun.

The truth is that supplements can play a supportive role in fertility. They work best when they are chosen with understanding rather than out of fear, pressure or comparison.

Most supplements used in fertility care support both egg and sperm health. A few are particularly important for women, such as folic acid, while others are sometimes added specifically to support sperm production. Please hold this in mind:

- You do not need everything you read about.
- You do not need the most expensive version of anything.
- You do not need to feel guilty if your supplement comes from a standard pharmacy or supermarket.
- Sometimes a supplement is helpful.
- Sometimes it is optional.
- And sometimes it is simply unnecessary.

Let's have a look at this in a little more detail.

Folic acid or methylfolate (for women)

Both folic acid and methylfolate support early embryo development and reduce the risk of neural tube defects. Folic acid is the standard form used in most UK supplements. Methylfolate is the active form, which some people absorb more easily. You do not need both.

Most people take 400 micrograms daily, which is the standard UK recommendation. Some individuals with higher BMI, diabetes or certain medical conditions may be advised to take 5mg daily, but in this case it is usually prescribed rather than bought over the counter.

> **Radical honesty: If you take only one supplement while trying to conceive, let it be folic acid.**

Vitamin D (for women and men)

Many people in the UK have low vitamin D, especially during autumn and winter. Low levels have been linked with hormonal imbalance, reduced implantation rates, lower IVF success and changes in mood. Vitamin D also plays a role in sperm production and overall reproductive hormone balance.

Most people are advised to take 10 micrograms (400IU) daily, which is the standard UK recommendation for adults. Some people with known deficiency or absorption issues may need higher doses, but this should be guided by a blood test or medical advice.

Omega 3 (fish oil or algae oil) (for women and men)

Omega 3 supports egg and sperm quality, hormone production, inflammation and early fetal development. If you do not regularly eat oily fish, a supplement can help.

CoQ10 (ubiquinol or ubiquinone) (for women and men)

Often suggested for those over 35 years of age or where egg or sperm quality is a concern, CoQ10 supports mitochondrial function, which is central to healthy egg and sperm development. Ubiquinol is more absorbable but more expensive. Ubiquinone is usually sufficient for most people.

CoQ10 is not essential for everyone, but it can be helpful in specific situations.

Inositol (primarily for women)

Inositol can help with ovulation, menstrual cycle regulation and egg quality and is often supportive for people with PMOS or insulin resistance. It is not needed unless clinically indicated.

Impryl (for women and men)

Impryl is slightly different. It does not behave like a typical antioxidant. Instead, it supports the body's own cellular repair pathways. It can be helpful in cases of sperm or egg DNA fragmentation, embryo quality issues or unexplained infertility. It is worth discussing with your medical team rather than buying automatically.

Additional supplements sometimes used to support sperm health (for men)

Other supplements that can help men include:

- Zinc
- Selenium
- Vitamins C and E
- L-carnitine

Your financial wellbeing matters too

This is worth stating clearly. There is a lot of noise around supplements, and it can create the impression that your fertility depends on having a long list of expensive products. That is not the case. A small number of evidence-based supplements can be genuinely helpful. The rest are optional, not essential.

Most of the meaningful gains do not come from supplements. They come from sleep, nourishment, lower alcohol intake, movement, emotional wellbeing and good clinical care.

If buying supplements creates financial pressure, that is a sign to step back rather than stretch yourself. You are not doing less. You are being sensible and protective of your wellbeing. Fertility does not improve because something costs more. It improves when your body feels supported in sustainable, realistic ways.

Staying organised with supplements

If you are taking supplements, you do not need to buy a weekly organiser to be a good patient. It is simply a practical tool that can make life easier if you find it hard to remember what you have taken. It reduces the mental load, supports consistency and removes the daily *Did I take that?* loop.

From here, we turn to the universal foundations that help both partners feel more prepared and better supported. The rest of the guidance applies to everyone, regardless of whether you are the one providing eggs or sperm. Gut health and everyday lifestyle factors influence the whole system, supporting hormone balance, inflammation, energy, immunity and the way in which your body responds to treatment.

Gut health

Gut health may not be the first thing you think of when preparing for fertility treatment, yet it plays a surprisingly meaningful role in how your body functions. Your gut microbiome influences inflammation, immune balance, hormone metabolism and how your body absorbs nutrients. These processes sit quietly in the background, but they help shape the internal environment needed for healthy menstrual cycles, implantation and overall reproductive wellbeing.

Emerging research continues to highlight how closely the gut is linked with reproductive health. A balanced gut can help regulate oestrogen, support progesterone, reduce low-grade inflammation and contribute to steadier energy and clearer digestion. None of this guarantees an outcome, but it strengthens the foundations on which your treatment will rely. Supporting your gut can be simple. You might include the following:

- Prebiotic foods such as garlic, onions, leeks, artichokes, asparagus, oats and bananas.
- Fermented foods such as live yoghurt, kefir, sauerkraut or kombucha.
- A wider variety of plant foods across the week.
- Fewer ultra-processed foods, which can create inflammation and disrupt microbial balance.

There is no need for strict rules or complicated routines. Small, consistent choices nourish the system that, in turn, supports your fertility. The same approach applies to lifestyle choices.

Lifestyle

Lifestyle is sometimes spoken about as if it is secondary to treatment, but in reality, it supports almost every process involved in fertility. Hormones, blood flow, sleep cycles, inflammation and even embryo development respond to how you live day to day.

Avoiding toxins

Sometimes, the most obvious things still need to be said plainly. Certain substances place real and unnecessary strain on egg and sperm development. Smoking and vaping can disrupt hormone balance and affect the DNA inside developing eggs and sperm. In women, recreational drugs and heavier alcohol use can interfere with ovulation, and in men, they can significantly reduce sperm motility and shape. Some workplaces also involve exposure to solvents, heat, pesticides or cytotoxic materials, which can quietly add to what your body is already managing.

You do not need to live a toxin-free life. You simply need to be aware of the exposures that matter most for fertility and reduce them where you can.

> **Radical honesty: Nicotine is one of the most damaging substances for fertility, and vaping is *not* a safer version. If you smoke or vape, stopping is one of the most powerful and impactful changes you can make for both egg and sperm health. This is not about criticism. It is about giving your body the best possible conditions to work well.**

Heat exposure

Heat can influence fertility more than people realise, especially in relation to sperm. Sperm are sensitive to temperature, and higher heat can affect their movement, shape and overall quality. Hot tubs, saunas, heated car seats, long cycling sessions, laptops resting on laps and very tight underwear can all raise scrotal temperature. The effects are usually reversible, but because sperm take around 90 days to mature, it is helpful to be mindful of heat in the months before treatment.

For women, the guidance is different. Daily life and warm baths are absolutely fine, but very high heat just before ovulation or embryo transfer is best avoided. Keeping the body warm is helpful. Raising internal temperature too much is not.

Movement and exercise

Movement plays an important role in fertility. It helps blood flow to the ovaries and testes, supports hormonal balance, steadies insulin levels and gently reduces inflammation. Even small amounts of movement can make your body feel more supported. What matters here is not the intensity but the steadiness and kindness of your approach.

For some people, exercise is a lifeline. It helps regulate mood, supports stress relief and offers a sense of routine. You do not need to give that up. You simply need to adapt so that your body feels cared for rather than depleted.

Gentle strength work, walking, swimming, stretching or yoga can all be helpful. These forms of movement encourage circulation without straining the body. As treatment progresses, especially during ovarian stimulation, the ovaries can become enlarged and tender. This is why high-impact exercise, twisting motions and anything that places pressure on the core are best avoided at this stage. Your goal is comfort, safety and support.

A helpful way to think about movement at this stage is to act as though you are already pregnant. If an activity would feel safe and comfortable in early pregnancy, it is usually a good guide for what is supportive now.

Avoiding extremes

Intense workouts, heavy lifting, high-intensity interval training and hot yoga can raise cortisol, disrupt hormonal rhythms and increase inflammation, especially during treatment cycles. These responses are natural, but they can add unnecessary stress to a system that is already working hard.

> **Radical honesty: This is not the season for chasing fitness milestones or working against your body. Choose the gentler version of whatever you normally do. Your body will recognise and appreciate the care.**

Let movement be something that helps you feel grounded rather than something you push yourself through. Caring for your body is never only about what you do. It is also about how you recover. Rest, especially the kind that comes through sleep, plays a central role in supporting fertility.

Sleep

Sleep supports almost every system involved in fertility. It helps regulate reproductive hormones, influences egg maturation, supports sperm development, reduces inflammation and strengthens the immune system. Many people are surprised by how closely their sleep patterns link with their menstrual cycles, mood and overall sense of wellbeing. Much of the body's repair work happens at night, which is why sleep is such a powerful part of preparation.

You may also find it helpful to learn your natural sleep rhythm if you do not already know it. Some people feel most awake and clear in the early morning and settle easily at night. Others find that their energy rises later in the day and they come alive in the evening. Neither pattern is right or wrong. What matters is working with your own biology rather than forcing yourself into a routine that suits other people. When you follow the rhythm that feels natural for your body, sleep often comes more easily and feels more restorative.

Good sleep is helped by simple habits that signal to your body that it is time to rest. This might include keeping a consistent bedtime where possible, dimming lights in the evening and allowing yourself a gradual wind-down rather than moving straight from activity to bed. A cool, quiet, dark room supports deeper rest, and leaving phones or laptops outside the bedroom can make it easier for your mind to settle. Many people find that a warm bath, light stretching, gentle reading or a calming routine helps the body shift into a different pace.

Small adjustments often make a bigger difference than people expect. Even one or two nights of deeper rest can shift how your body feels and how well it responds to the demands of treatment.

Radical honesty: Improving your sleep may be one of the most meaningful things you can do for your fertility.

Once the lifestyle foundations we've discussed so far are in place, some people choose to add therapies that offer a different kind of support. These are optional, not essential, but they can sit alongside treatment in a way that feels steady and regulating. One of the most commonly used therapies is acupuncture.

Acupuncture

Acupuncture is often used alongside fertility treatment. It is not a replacement for medical care, but it can support the body in several ways that matter during treatment. What the evidence suggests:

- It can improve blood flow to the uterus and ovaries, which may support the development of the uterine lining.
- It may help regulate the hormones that influence ovulation and menstrual cycles.
- It can reduce stress hormones and support the parasympathetic nervous system (the body's rest and recovery system).
- Some studies suggest it may improve IVF outcomes, particularly around embryo transfer, though findings vary.

If you choose to try acupuncture, consistency matters more than perfect timing. Many people find it most supportive in the weeks leading up to stimulation and during the calmer days between appointments. Choose a practitioner with experience in fertility care. They will understand treatment cycle timing, stimulation protocols and clinic guidelines.

Acupuncture can be helpful, but it is not essential. Some people find it calming and regulating. Others prefer not to add additional appointments during an already demanding time. Both choices are valid.

While acupuncture is something you may choose to include, the environment you live and work in affects you every day, often without you noticing. What you breathe in, what touches your skin, what you store food in and what you're exposed to at work all play a role in reproductive health. You do not need to control everything, but understanding the small adjustments that genuinely help can reduce unnecessary strain on your body.

Environment

When it comes to environment and fertility, people are often given mixed messages. Some clinics ask women not to wear perfume or scented products on the day of egg collection or embryo transfer, which can understandably make you worry about everything you put on your skin or bring into your home. It can feel as though every product needs scrutiny, which is both overwhelming and unnecessary.

The evidence tells us something simpler. Certain chemicals can interfere with hormones when exposure is high or prolonged. These are called endocrine-disrupting chemicals, and they are found in a range of everyday products, from some plastics to heavy fragrances to certain cleaning agents. They do not need to be eliminated entirely. What helps is reducing unnecessary exposure where it is easy and realistic to do so.

Clinics ask you to avoid perfume on procedure days because strong fragrances contain volatile compounds that can affect air quality in small theatre spaces and embryology laboratories. This is a very specific request for a very controlled environment. It does not mean that occasional perfume use is a proven cause of fertility problems in everyday life.

If you want to make gentle, evidence-based changes, these are the ones that tend to matter:

- Choose fragrance-free or low-fragrance cleaning products where possible.

- Use glass or stainless steel for food storage instead of very old or damaged plastic.
- Avoid heating food in plastic containers.
- Improve ventilation by opening windows or using an extractor fan.
- Consider a simple water filter if your area has hard water or older pipes.
- Be mindful of strong chemical exposures (especially solvents or pesticides) in certain workplaces.

These adjustments reduce background exposure in a kind, sustainable way. They do not demand a toxin-free home. Most importantly, they help you feel more informed and less anxious. You can make changes without entering the world of extremes.

> **Radical honesty: You are not harming your fertility by wearing moisturiser, using shampoo or applying your usual skincare. What matters is thoughtful reduction of the exposures that genuinely influence reproductive health. Small steps are enough.**

Our environment also shapes our mental and emotional approach to this journey far more than most people discuss openly. We discuss these aspects in the second part of this chapter (*see* pp. 137–51).

Fertility at work

Treatment does not pause for meetings, deadlines or inboxes. You may find yourself organising scans around work hours, taking calls in private, injecting yourself in the bathroom or trying to concentrate while waiting for results. None of this is small or easy to manage. In fact, holding together your professional life and treatment at the same time can be exhausting.

Some people choose to tell their workplace; others keep it private. There is no right or wrong approach here, only the one that protects your sense of safety. In the UK, there is no specific legal entitlement to fertility leave at the time of writing, but many workplaces offer flexibility through sick days, annual leave or remote working. You might choose to speak with HR, a trusted manager or one supportive colleague so you are not carrying the weight alone. Supportive approaches might include:

- Planning lighter workloads during stimulation.
- Arranging remote days or flexible hours where possible.

- Scheduling injections or rest breaks when you can.
- Taking space after difficult appointments.
- Holding compassion for tiredness and limited focus.

Needing flexibility does not make you less committed, nor is it a reflection of you or your ability to do your job.

As you can see, the physical foundations of fertility preparation are practical, grounded and largely within your influence. Nutrition, movement, sleep, metabolic health, environmental exposures and lifestyle choices all help create the conditions in which hormones regulate, eggs and sperm mature and treatment medications work as they are designed to. None of these steps guarantee an outcome, but they do support the systems your body relies on during fertility treatment.

It is also important to remember that preparation does not mean perfection. You are not being asked to follow every suggestion or create an idealised version of health. Small, steady changes tend to be far more supportive than rigid rules or sudden overhauls. The aim is not control, but support.

Yet fertility treatment does not unfold only within the body. It unfolds within a mind that is constantly making sense of what is happening. Thoughts, emotions, expectations and uncertainty all move alongside the physical process. While caring for your body creates an important foundation, caring for your mind can make the journey itself feel steadier and more manageable.

With that in mind, we now turn to the second part of this chapter: how to care for your emotional world as you move through fertility treatment.

Part 2: caring for your mind

This part of the chapter will help you consider how your inner world responds to treatment. Not just the obvious feelings like hope and fear, but the quieter ones too: uncertainty, comparison, frustration, tenderness, anticipation and the in-between state that fertility treatment often brings. You are not being asked to become emotionally perfect or endlessly calm. You are being invited to understand what supports you, what helps you stay connected to yourself and what makes this process more manageable.

Although fertility treatment is a medical pathway, it unfolds inside a living, thinking, feeling human being: you. This is not about blame, resilience myths or the idea that you must think positively to conceive.

Instead, we explore where gentle psychological support can soften the edges of treatment and help it feel less lonely.

Preparing your mind is not about eliminating difficult feelings. It is about creating room for them without being swept away, finding ways to soothe yourself and building anchors you can return to. These foundations do not remove uncertainty, but they can make the process more bearable, more humane and more within your sense of control.

EXERCISE: CONTROLLING THE CONTROLLABLES

This exercise is designed to bring clarity to the fertility process, which can sometimes feel chaotic. When you gently separate what sits within your influence from what does not, something begins to settle. The aim is to help you feel a greater sense of direction and agency as you move forwards.

Step one
Take a piece of paper and draw a line down the middle. Label one side 'Within my control' and the other 'Outside my control'.

Step two
Begin with the 'Outside my control' column. Write down the parts of treatment or life that you cannot direct, predict or guarantee. Keep it brief. A few key items are enough.

Step three
Move to the 'Within my control' column. Add the areas where your choices, boundaries or habits genuinely make a difference. Again, keep it simple.

Step four
Look at both lists together. Notice any small shift in how you feel. Many people describe having a little more space, or the sense that the process is slightly easier to hold.

Step five
Choose one item from the 'Within my control' list and ask yourself: *What is one small thing I can do this week to support myself here?* **There is no right answer, only what feels possible for you.**

Stress and fertility: understanding what really matters

Stress is one of the most misunderstood parts of fertility. Many people quietly worry that feeling anxious, overwhelmed or emotional will reduce their chances of conceiving. Some try to stay endlessly calm. Others blame themselves for every moment of worry, as if a single anxious thought could alter an outcome.

That is a heavy burden to carry. And it is also *not true*.

Human beings have conceived, carried and birthed babies through every imaginable version of stress: war, famine, migration, grief, poverty, illness, heartbreak and profound uncertainty. It is simply not biologically plausible that everyday stress would prevent conception in an otherwise healthy system.

Where stress becomes relevant is not in feeling it but in how you are forced to hold it. There is a difference between stress that moves through the body and stress that becomes trapped because it has nowhere to go. When stress is acknowledged, spoken about, shared, understood or supported, it tends to ease. The body finds ways to regulate. Hormones settle. Sleep improves. Muscles soften. The system rebalances. When stress is pushed down or hidden because you feel you must stay positive or composed, the body absorbs it. This is the difference between everyday stress and the heavy, internalised burden described in trauma research. What affects fertility is not the presence of stress itself but the chronic, unprocessed strain that builds when you suppress what you feel or try to cope entirely alone.

It is our fundamental belief that stress becomes easier for the body to manage when you take these steps:

- Speak gently about what feels difficult.
- Let someone sit with you in your worry.
- Allow your emotions to surface rather than tighten around them.
- Rest when you are depleted.
- Use grounding practices that bring you back into the present moment.
- Reach for support rather than withdrawing.

These are the moments when your system recalibrates.

Radical honesty: Feeling stressed does not mean you are harming your fertility. What harms you is carrying everything inside without support. Stress that is shared, felt, named and softened through connection is entirely compatible with fertility.

This is where emotional anchors come in. They give your system places to land when things feel uncertain. They help you feel accompanied rather than overwhelmed. They make it easier to be with your real experience instead of fighting it internally.

What we mean by 'anchors'

When we use the word anchors in this book, we are referring to small, grounding practices that help you return to yourself when the process feels overwhelming. Anchors can be moments, rituals, pauses or habits that give your nervous system something familiar and steady to lean on. They remind your body that it is not under threat, even when things feel emotionally charged.

> **Radical honesty: When you acknowledge your inner experience rather than pushing it away, something settles inside you.**

Examples of emotional anchors

- A quiet check-in with yourself at the beginning or end of the day.
- A slow breathing practice that softens your body.
- A few written lines that help clear your mind.
- A gentle walk to reconnect with the world around you.
- A grounding phrase that brings you back into the moment.
- A weekly check-in with your partner or someone you trust.
- Allowing yourself to rest on difficult days.
- Protecting your emotional energy with simple boundaries.

These do not remove uncertainty; they help you stand more steadily within it. And of all the things you will meet on this journey, uncertainty is one of the hardest to hold.

Living with uncertainty

If one thing is certain in fertility, it is that you will meet uncertainty. You may not know how long things will take or how you will respond. You may not know what tomorrow's appointment will bring. This lack of clarity can feel unsettling, because you are dealing with something tender and deeply important.

It is natural to want answers, and it is natural to want clear timelines. Yet much of fertility cannot be predicted with precision. What can steady you is not certainty but agency.

This means that even when outcomes are unknown, you still have meaningful ways to participate. You can ask questions, request clear explanations from your clinic, take notes and rest when your mind feels full. These are not small acts; they are there to reinforce your place within your own story.

Examples of uncertainty anchors

- Preparing one or two questions before each appointment.
- Asking for simple language to be used when medical explanations become overwhelming.
- Focusing on the next step rather than the entire journey.
- Pausing after appointments to let information settle.
- Limiting the number of websites you consult.
- Saying to yourself: 'I do not have to know everything today.'

Accepting uncertainty means directing your energy towards what is yours to hold and letting the rest fall away. It is a quiet recognition of what is within your control and what is not, and allowing yourself to release the parts that were never yours to manage. Once you understand this, you can begin to build resilience.

Understanding resilience

What does resilience mean to you? Over the years, we have heard many people speak about resilience as if it means holding everything together – not crying, not complaining and never showing fear – as though strength is measured by how tightly you can control your emotions. These beliefs run deep, especially around fertility, where people often feel they must stay strong at all times to cope or to deserve progress.

But none of this is true.

Resilience is not about staying positive or keeping everything neatly in place. Real resilience is flexible and human, allowing you to feel deeply and still find your way back to yourself. It makes room for tiredness and fear, for frustration as well as hope, and it bends with you rather than asking you to stay upright at every moment.

Support is part of resilience. In fact, it is one of its foundations. You are not meant to move through this alone. Partners, friends, therapists, support groups and cultural or faith communities can help hold what feels too heavy for one person.

Examples of resilience anchors

- Resting without guilt.
- Reaching for support rather than enduring alone.
- Returning to simple grounding practices when emotions rise.
- Allowing yourself to pause before making decisions.
- Speaking kindly to yourself in moments of doubt.
- Keeping small rituals that offer comfort.

These practices do not remove difficulty, but they hopefully make it liveable. And at the heart of resilience is one essential skill: self-compassion.

Self-compassion

Sadly, in our experience, fertility challenges often bring a quiet sense of shame. Shame about not performing in the way you think you should. Shame about not coping as well as others imagine you are. Shame about your body not responding as expected, or about feeling emotions you believe you ought to have outgrown. This shame is heavy, and it is misplaced and undeserved.

There will be days when you feel capable and hopeful, and days when you feel tired, unsure or overwhelmed by the pace of the process. You may have moments when you feel disappointed with your body or frustrated by the waiting. These feelings are part of being human in the middle of something deeply important.

The antidote to shame is self-compassion. Self-compassion is not indulgence; it is a form of medicine. Self-compassion softens the harshness that people so often direct towards themselves. It makes space for rest when you are tired, for asking for help when you need it and for feeling your emotions without turning them into evidence of failure. It creates pockets of gentleness in the middle of uncertainty, allowing moments of joy to exist even when life feels complicated.

A SELF-COMPASSION EXERCISE: SPEAKING TO YOURSELF AS YOU WOULD SPEAK TO A FRIEND

Find a quiet place where you can sit comfortably. Let your body settle. You may want to place a hand on your chest or your lap to remind you that you are here, in this moment, and that you matter.

Step one

Think of someone you care about. Someone whose pain you would never dismiss and whose feelings you would treat with softness. Imagine that this person is sitting in front of you, telling you about the very thing you are struggling with today. Perhaps they feel disappointed with their body. Perhaps they are tired of waiting. Perhaps they are frightened about what lies ahead.

Step two

Notice, gently, what rises in you. Most people find compassion almost instantly. Kindness. Understanding. A desire to reassure. We rarely judge the people we love for their pain. We meet them with warmth, because we want them to feel supported rather than alone.

Step three

Now imagine directing those same words, that same tone, towards yourself. You do not need to force it. Just try. What would you say if you spoke to yourself the way you speak to someone you care for deeply? You might say:

- 'I know this is hard.'
- 'You are doing the best you can.'
- 'It makes sense that you feel this way.'
- 'You deserve rest.'
- 'You are allowed to soften.'
- 'You do not have to carry this alone.'

Let the words land gently. They do not need to fix anything. Their purpose is simply to ease the tightness that shame and self-criticism create.

Step four

Take one slow breath. Notice any small shift, even if it is subtle. Self-compassion is a practice, not a performance. It becomes easier with repetition.

When you treat yourself with the same tenderness you offer others, something inside you begins to settle. You may not feel instantly better, but you will feel more connected to yourself, and that connection is one of the most protective things you can offer your emotional wellbeing.

Radical honesty: You are more than a fertility diagnosis or treatment. You are a whole person with a whole life. You deserve connection, tenderness and meaning – not later when this is over, but now, exactly as you are.

From this place of gentleness and honesty, we can turn towards the deeper truth that sits beneath this journey: radical honesty, and what that really means.

Radical honesty

There is a quiet truth at the heart of emotional suffering: much of the pain we feel does not come from the emotion itself but from the struggle against it. The effort to push away sadness. The determination to hide fear. The pressure to stay positive when we feel anything but. The belief that we should be coping better than we are.

Radical honesty: Emotional suffering often comes from resisting what is.

When we refuse our experience, it tightens, and the fear grows. The sadness may deepen, and the frustration sometimes becomes heavier. Not because the feeling is wrong, but because we are fighting our own reality. Radical honesty is the gentle act of stopping that fight.

It means acknowledging what is already true, even if you wish it were different. This is hard! It asks for courage. But naming your experience does not make it worse. In fact, it does the opposite: it makes it more bearable. It turns emotional chaos into something you can sit with, something you can understand, something you can soothe. Radical honesty may sound like this:

- 'This is hard for me.'
- 'I am scared today.'
- 'I feel hopeful and anxious at the same time.'
- 'I am tired.'
- 'I need help.'
- 'I am grieving something I cannot fully name.'
- 'I wish this were easier.'

When you allow your experience to exist, rather than resisting or hiding it, your emotional system can settle. You may not feel instantly calm, but you will feel a little more in control. The suffering eases because the struggle eases.

Radical honesty is about meeting yourself as you are, so that you can move through what comes next with clarity, dignity and self-respect. Honesty brings clarity, and clarity often shows us where we may need extra care. This is where therapy can offer a steady and compassionate space to hold what feels too heavy to carry alone.

Therapy and support

Therapy can be one of the most supportive parts of fertility care. It offers a private space where you can speak openly without needing to stay strong or make sense of everything on your own.

Therapy is not a sign of weakness. It is a sign that you are taking your emotional wellbeing seriously. It helps you process what is happening, understand your reactions and find steadier ground when things feel overwhelming.

It can also support your relationship. Fertility challenges place pressure on communication, often in ways couples do not expect. A therapeutic space helps you talk honestly, understand each other's needs and stay connected through a demanding time.

Therapy sits alongside everyday support rather than replacing it. Small practices and simple moments of care can help you stay grounded between appointments and give you ways of looking after yourself when emotions shift.

FINDING THE RIGHT THERAPIST FOR YOU

You do not need to stay with the first therapist you find. The fit really does matter, and so does the sense of rapport you have with them. A therapeutic relationship should feel safe and steady. It should be a place where you can talk freely and feel understood, not a space you have to push yourself into or perform within. If you sense something is off, you are allowed to keep looking until you find someone who feels like the right match for you.

It is also important that your therapist understands fertility. Without that expertise, sessions can drift into explaining scans, medications, timelines and procedures rather than exploring how all of this is impacting you. The right therapist already knows the landscape you are walking through, which means the session time is spent on your emotional world, not on filling gaps in their knowledge.

Therapy can offer a place to speak freely and feel understood, but support does not end when the session finishes. There are small, everyday practices that help you stay connected to yourself between conversations, especially when emotions rise or decisions accumulate. One of the simplest and most helpful of these is mindfulness.

Mindfulness

Mindfulness is the practice of bringing yourself back to the present moment. Not to clear your mind or silence your thoughts, but simply to notice what is there with a little more softness and a little less judgement. It is a way of offering your nervous system a brief pause when everything feels full.

It can be as simple as slowing your breath, feeling the weight of your feet on the floor, resting your hand on your chest, noticing the temperature of the air around you, or pausing at the window for a moment before returning to your day. These small acts can create tiny pockets of calm that help your body settle.

Mindfulness does not require long meditation sessions or a perfect technique. It is made up of brief, ordinary moments where you come back to yourself. A single slow breath. A gentle stretch. A pause before you speak. A moment of noticing the sensations in your body rather than rushing past them.

A MINDFULNESS EXERCISE

Find a comfortable position, either sitting or standing. Let your shoulders drop a little, and allow your hands to rest wherever they naturally fall.

Step one

Take one slow breath in through your nose, and let the exhale be just a little longer than the inhale. You do not need to change anything about your breathing after this. Just notice it.

▶

Step two

Bring your attention to the contact your body is making with the ground or the chair. Notice the weight in your feet, your legs and your back. You are simply observing, not trying to feel anything in particular.

Step three

Gently widen your awareness. Notice three things you can feel in your body. Warmth. Coolness. Clothing against your skin. The movement of your breath. Let these sensations be exactly as they are.

Step four

If your mind wanders, that is completely normal. When you notice it, guide your attention back to your breath or the feeling of your feet on the floor. There is no right way to do this. You are simply practising returning to yourself.

Step five

Take one more slow breath. When you are ready, allow your attention to come back to the room around you. Notice any small shift in your body, even if it is very subtle.

This exercise takes less than a minute, but it can bring a gentle sense of steadiness into moments that feel rushed or overwhelming. You can use it before an appointment, after a phone call, while waiting for results or simply when you need a pause.

Environment

Mindfulness practices do not remove stress, but they hopefully soften its grip. With this, we can also speak honestly about what helps and does not help in relation to your environment. Fertility treatment does not happen in isolation. It lives inside your daily interactions, your rhythms as a couple, work schedules, bank accounts, family expectations, social invitations and the reality of everyday life. Many people tell us that it is not only the injections or the waiting that feels hard, but the weight of trying to hold everything else at the same time. We therefore conclude our guide to caring for your mind by exploring these external environmental pressures.

Money and relationships

The financial side of treatment can place pressure on relationships in ways that many couples do not expect. It is common for one partner to feel anxious about the cost, while the other feels desperate to continue. One person may want to take a break, while the other is afraid to lose time. These tensions do not mean the relationship is weak. They mean the stakes are high and the emotional weight is real.

When couples talk openly about money, something often softens. Not because the situation becomes easier, but because the pressure becomes shared rather than carried alone. It can help to sit together and gently explore:

- How far you feel comfortable going financially.
- What level of debt feels manageable rather than frightening.
- Whether help from family is welcome or would create pressure.
- What might bring peace if treatment takes longer than hoped.

We have found that some couples find relief in setting a financial boundary together. For some people, family can offer financial help. For others, support is not available, or it is offered with expectations attached. Each situation carries its own emotional complexity, like most family dynamics.

Financial planning is about reducing uncertainty in a process that already holds so much of it. You might choose to prepare for one treatment cycle at a time or create a plan that considers the possibility of more. You may decide to take a break to restore yourselves emotionally or financially. Try to approach this part of the journey in the same way you approach treatment itself. One appointment at a time. One payment at a time. One conversation at a time.

Sex, intimacy and connection

Fertility treatment can change the way in which we experience sex, sometimes suddenly and sometimes gradually. Hormones may shift desire. Physical discomfort may make intimacy feel different. Scan schedules, medications and the emotional weight of the process can place a quiet strain on how connected you feel to your own body and to your partner. None of this is a sign that something is wrong; instead, it is a reflection of your body and mind responding to a demanding season.

Closeness does not need to disappear when sex feels different. It can simply shift. Many couples find it helpful to focus on forms of connection that feel comfortable and manageable during treatment. This might include sitting close while watching something together, holding hands, sharing a meal without phones, going for a short walk or having small check-in conversations at the end of the day. Some couples schedule a weekly moment of connection, which can even be just 10 minutes to talk about something other than treatment. Others create simple rituals, like making morning coffee for each other or maintaining a shared routine that brings steadiness. These are practical ways to keep intimacy alive when sex feels pressured or physically uncomfortable.

> **Radical honesty: Fertility treatment can temporarily change how you feel in your body, and for many people this arrives as an unspoken loss. Sometimes, the softest and most helpful thing you can do is name it gently to yourself or to your partner. Naming it often brings relief.**

Family, friends and social life

You may want people around you, you may find that you want privacy or you may want both at different times. Fertility is emotionally complex, and your needs may shift over time and even day to day. It can help to decide who you want to tell and in what amount, and what kind of support feels nourishing rather than draining.

Support can look like any of these scenarios:

- One trusted friend you can message after appointments.
- Family members who step in when you need rest.
- A colleague who discreetly covers a meeting.
- Someone who will listen without offering solutions.

Boundaries can look like this:

- Saying no to baby-centred events.
- Asking not to be asked for updates.
- Leaving early when conversations become painful.
- Choosing silence some days and connection on others.

You do not have to be available to every space or every person. Protecting your energy is part of caring for yourself.

Toxic positivity

In the UK, there is often a quiet expectation that we will stay positive, keep calm and carry on, even when life feels anything but calm. People may encourage you to look on the bright side, to stay hopeful, to keep smiling, to trust the process. Most of this is well meant, yet it can leave you feeling unseen, especially when your emotional world is more complex than the words people offer you.

Fertility can stir many emotions. You may move between sadness, hope, fear, frustration and gratitude in a single week. These shifts do not mean you are losing perspective. They reflect the intensity and uncertainty of what you are moving through.

Forced positivity can become a kind of emotional silencing. When you feel pressure to appear strong or cheerful, the emotions that need most care are often the ones you push down. This can leave you feeling even more alone.

What helps is not constant optimism but honesty. Gentleness. Permission to feel what is true for you without trying to make it more palatable for others.

We also know that the people around you may not always know what to say or do. Many want to be supportive but worry about saying the wrong thing. Fertility treatment can be difficult for others to understand, especially if they have not experienced it themselves. You may find that some people are incredibly thoughtful, while others feel unsure or unintentionally say things that miss the mark.

You do not need to carry the responsibility of educating everyone around you. It is reasonable to ask for the support you need, to set gentle boundaries where necessary and to share as much or as little about your experience as feels right for you.

Radical honesty: Fertility can make people uncomfortable. When people feel uncomfortable, they often try to fix, minimise or move past the feeling rather than sit with it. That discomfort belongs to them, not to you. It is not your job to make everyone else comfortable. Your priority is caring for yourself.

Living in a pronatal culture

You may notice pregnancy announcements appearing around you without warning. You might sit through conversations about feeding routines or nursery choices and feel yourself drifting inside.

It is okay if joy for others sits alongside a sort of sadness and sometimes bitterness for yourself. Here are some gentle reminders that may help:

- You are not behind, even if it feels like it.
- You are not less than, because this is hard.
- You are allowed to step back when needed.
- You do not owe anyone constant emotional strength.

It can also bring emotions that feel uncomfortable to admit out loud, jealousy, envy, resentment or even anger towards people whose lives seem to be moving forward while yours feels painfully stuck. You may find yourself avoiding baby announcements, struggling at children's birthdays or feeling disconnected from friends who are pregnant. These reactions can make people feel guilty or ashamed, but they are far more common than most people realise. Difficult emotions do not make you a bad person. They are often a reflection of grief, exhaustion and longing colliding all at once.

A closing reflection

As you prepare emotionally, begin to notice the quieter shifts taking place within you. You are building a foundation that is not simply about coping but also about meeting this journey with clarity and self-awareness. Preparation does not follow a straight line, and it certainly does not look the same for everyone. There is no single right way to do this. There is only the way that fits your temperament, your history, your values and the pace at which you feel able to move.

Try to care for your mind with the same attentiveness you offer your body. Let support in when it reaches towards you. Speak to yourself in a tone you would recognise as fair, thoughtful and kind. And allow your emotions to exist without rushing them or dressing them up.

You are taking deliberate steps towards something that holds meaning for you. Those steps may feel small or uneven at times, but they are steps all the same. For now, let it be enough that you are moving forward with intention and care.

Reflective questions

Take a moment here to think about the following questions:

- What emotions are present in me today, and what might they be asking for?

- Where do I already feel supported, and where might I want more support?
- Which small practices help me return to myself?
- What helps me feel grounded when I do not have answers?
- What boundaries would support my emotional wellbeing?
- What would it look like to meet this next stage with gentleness rather than pressure?

Final thoughts

We have witnessed how many people approach fertility treatment with an unspoken pressure to get everything right. The perfect diet. The perfect supplements. The perfect emotional state. Yet perfection is not what supports you. What supports you is a conscious and kind way of caring for yourself.

When we speak about a conscious approach, we mean something simple and human. Noticing how you move through your days. Noticing how you rest, how you speak to yourself, how you allow your emotional life to matter.

The second part is kindness: a quality that softens the edges of a demanding process. Kindness allows you to pause. It allows you to meet your experience with compassion rather than criticism. It reminds you that you deserve gentleness even in a time that asks so much of you.

This way of approaching treatment is not about controlling the outcome. It is about controlling the environment you create inside yourself as you move forward. A conscious and kind approach makes room for your whole self. It is one of the greatest acts of self-compassion you can offer yourself during this journey.

In chapter 7, we will walk through what IVF treatments look like in everyday life, step by step, so that when you are ready, you can continue with clarity, confidence and support.

7

Seven key stages of IVF:

what to expect and when

Before we go anywhere near needles, timings, scans or numbers, we want to begin with you.

If you were sitting with us right now, we would not start by listing medications or explaining protocols. We would begin with reassurance. We would begin by helping you feel seen, and helping you feel that you will be supported throughout the process. IVF asks a great deal of your body, your time and your emotional capacity. IVF is complex, but preparation helps. We hope that a clear understanding of what lies ahead turns a confusing process into one you can approach with more certainty and control.

So, when you are ready, we will move through this chapter stage by stage. Perhaps first, take a moment and notice where you are. Curious? Nervous? Hopeful? Exhausted? Maybe a little of each? Whatever shows up, meet it with kindness. You are allowed to be exactly where you are.

IVF can feel like a world of its own. The language is unfamiliar, the process can appear clinical and complex and it is common to wonder how you will cope or whether any of this will work. If you notice those thoughts, you are not alone in them.

Before we go further, here are three simple truths:

- You do not have to understand everything right now.
- You do not have to remember every step.
- You only need to take this one stage at a time.

The intention here is to make the process understandable and manageable, so you can move through it with more confidence.

Why this chapter focuses on IVF

There are a few reasons to go more in-depth with IVF treatment (chapter 8 covers the other types of fertility treatment you may encounter). IVF is the treatment many people eventually meet, either in the NHS or privately, because it offers the highest success rates among assisted fertility treatments when first-line approaches have not led to pregnancy. It is also the treatment with the most clearly defined stages. By understanding IVF, you begin to understand many of the medicines, tests and decisions that appear in other treatments too. The same hormones, scans and clinical choices often appear in adapted forms across other pathways, which means learning about IVF gives you a foundation that translates beyond this chapter.

We will walk you through the seven key stages of IVF. We will begin with preparation and stimulation, move into egg and sperm collection, follow the embryos as they grow in the laboratory and then arrive at transfer and the waiting days that follow. We will finish at test day and explore what may come next. At each stage, we will look at both what happens medically and what this experience can feel like in everyday life.

IVF in simple terms

At its most basic, IVF means that eggs are collected from your body and fertilised with sperm in a laboratory, then the resulting embryos are transferred into the uterus.

That is the medical description. It is accurate but incomplete.

IVF is not only a medical process, it is also a deeply emotional and vulnerable experience. It asks for time, patience, physical energy and a willingness to keep hoping in the face of uncertainty. IVF can change your daily routine, your sleep, your relationship with your body and sometimes your sense of yourself.

Let us begin at the point where IVF begins to shape everyday life in a practical way.

Stage one: preparation and ovarian stimulation

This is where IVF begins to feel real. The ovarian stimulation phase (*see* pp. 215–17) is also the most physically demanding stage, as your body is working harder now, and you may start to notice the process in a more tangible sense.

Before the stimulation itself, you will usually have a planning appointment and baseline tests. These might include blood tests, internal scans, semen analysis (*see* pp. 83–85) and a conversation about your personalised treatment plan and protocol (*see* chapter 10).

> **Radical honesty: Most scans during IVF are internal, even if you have your period. This may feel uncomfortable at first, but it is standard practice, and your clinicians should treat it with care and professionalism. You can ask for a chaperone, bring a support person or say that you feel nervous. Your comfort matters.**

Once your plan is agreed, stimulation begins. The purpose here is to encourage your ovaries to develop more follicles than they would in a natural cycle, so that several eggs can be collected rather than just one. In the laboratory, each egg will have its own journey. Some will fertilise; others may not. Some embryos will continue to grow; others may slow or stop. This is part of the biology of reproduction, both inside and outside the body. When there are multiple eggs to work with, you create more opportunities for one embryo to develop in a way that could lead to transfer and, with time, perhaps a pregnancy.

Daily life during stimulation

During stimulation you will usually take hormone injections once or twice a day for around eight to fourteen days. These medicines encourage your ovaries to grow follicles, which are the fluid-filled sacs that hold eggs. You will have regular monitoring appointments during this stage. Most clinics scan every two or three days to check how many follicles are growing and how quickly they are developing. You may also have blood tests to look at your hormone levels, particularly oestradiol, which rises as follicles mature. These pieces of information together show whether the ovaries are responding as expected. The clinic are looking for the following:

- How many follicles are developing.
- Whether they are growing at a healthy pace.
- Whether your hormone levels match what they are seeing on the scan.
- Whether your medication dose needs adjusting.

- When you are approaching the point where a trigger injection (*see* pp. 159–61) can be scheduled.

Medication doses are sometimes changed during this stage. This does not mean something is wrong. It means your team are tailoring treatment in real time to support your body. As your body responds, the clinic responds to your body.

These appointments are often early in the morning so that people can get to work afterwards. Even so, IVF can begin to shape the rhythm of daily life. There may be a need to consider travel, parking, waiting, fitting appointments around jobs, childcare or routines and the quiet background thought of when the next injection or scan is due. Many people describe this stage as living life around a timetable.

Physically, treatment looks different for everyone. You may feel bloated or full in your lower abdomen as follicles grow. You might notice tenderness around the injection sites or find yourself moving more slowly because your ovaries are working hard. Some days, you may feel fine. Other days, you may feel tired or fed up. It is all part of your body responding to stimulation.

A note on the physical side

Stimulation asks a great deal of your body. Your ovaries are growing multiple follicles rather than just one, and that takes physical space as well as energy. You may feel heavy through your lower abdomen, bloated in a way that means clothes feel tighter or aware of your pelvic area in a way you never usually are. Headaches, fatigue and a sense of fullness are also common. Some people describe feeling slowed down or unsettled in their bodies for a little while.

This does not mean something is wrong. It is simply what it feels like when the ovaries are working harder than usual. You can always ask your clinic how to manage discomfort, and if anything feels sharp, severe or worrying, it is reasonable to seek advice.

Radical honesty: You do not have to be positive every day. Treatment can feel tiring, boring, inconvenient or unfair.

As follicles grow, your clinic will watch for the point where they are ready. Before we move on to the trigger injection and egg collection, it is important to talk about safety during stimulation, because this is when the ovaries are most active and most sensitive to hormone changes.

Ovarian hyperstimulation syndrome (OHSS)

A small number of people develop OHSS. OHSS happens when the ovaries respond very strongly to medication and produce a high number of follicles, causing fluid to move into the abdomen. This can lead to swelling, discomfort and, in more severe cases, shortness of breath or nausea. Your clinic will monitor closely for this throughout stimulation, and modern IVF protocols are designed to reduce the risk wherever possible.

Some people are more likely to develop OHSS, including those with a high ovarian reserve or with PMOS (*see* pp. 30–31). If this applies to you, your clinic may use a gentler approach to stimulation or choose a different trigger medication to keep you safe. Prevention is a key part of care.

Mild symptoms might include:

- Bloating or abdominal discomfort.
- Feeling full quickly.
- Mild nausea.

More concerning symptoms include:

- Rapid abdominal swelling.
- Shortness of breath.
- Severe pain.
- Vomiting.
- Reduced urine output.

As your oestrogen levels rise during the stimulation phase and your eggs begin to develop, your body will naturally draw in water, which you will need to replenish. The more follicles you have, the more water your body requires. It is essential that your clinic monitors your hydration levels and asks about your fluid intake. If they have not addressed this, do not hesitate to raise the question yourself.

TOP TIPS

- Please aim to drink a glass of fluid every hour while you are awake. It makes it much easier to hit the amount your body needs to stay supported. Carry a bottle everywhere. Yes, you'll be running to the toilet a lot, but it's essential.

- Eating every two to three hours is just as important. Some people find they feel too full from the fluids alone, which is why 'small and often' really matters.

Focus on a high-protein diet (*see* below) where you can, as it helps your body manage the fluid shifts between cells and can ease the bloating.

How protein supports your body during stimulation

Protein plays an important role during IVF, particularly in managing bloating and fluid balance. Inside the bloodstream, a protein called albumin helps to hold fluid inside the blood vessels. When albumin levels are healthy, fluid is more likely to stay where it is needed rather than leaking into the tissues. If protein intake is low, albumin can drop and fluid may escape more easily. This is when bloating and abdominal heaviness can feel more intense.

During IVF, rising hormones can make the blood vessels more porous. Fluid may move into the belly or tissues, which is what creates swelling and that tight, stretched feeling. A higher protein intake supports albumin production, helping the body keep fluid where it belongs. Alongside staying well hydrated, this can reduce discomfort and help you feel steadier in your body as treatment continues. Adequate protein intake has a number of benefits:

- Your body can produce more albumin.
- More fluid stays within the blood vessels.
- Less fluid leaks into the surrounding tissues.
- Bloating is often reduced.
- Stimulation may feel easier to tolerate.

For this reason, many clinics recommend increasing protein intake during stimulation and after egg collection, especially if you are at higher risk of bloating or OHSS (*see* p. 157).

Helpful sources include eggs, chicken, fish, tofu, lentils, Greek yoghurt, quinoa and beans. Some people also use protein shakes if appetite is low or meals are difficult to manage. This is not about extreme eating but about offering your body enough support to handle the fluid shifts that hormones can create.

When the follicles reach the right size and your hormone levels suggest they are nearly mature, your clinic will arrange the next step. This is the trigger injection, which prepares the eggs for collection.

Stage two: trigger injection and egg collection

When your follicles have grown to a point where they appear ready, your clinic will let you know it is time for the trigger injection (*see* pp. 159–61), so that eggs can be collected. This final medicine helps the eggs complete their maturation so they can be collected during the procedure that follows. Timing matters here. The injection needs to be taken when the clinic advises, so the eggs are ready but not yet released.

> **Radical honesty: The timing of the trigger can feel intense. You may be asked to take it at a very specific hour, sometimes even down to the minute. When you are tired or emotional, this can feel like a lot to hold. Many people set multiple alarms, write down the instructions more than once or ask someone to be with them when the time comes. This is not overcaution. It is care.**

After your trigger injection, egg collection is usually planned for around 35–37 hours later. This is the window in which the eggs are mature and accessible, and in which your clinic will guide you into the next stage.

Egg collection day

Egg collection usually takes place under sedation. You will be asleep or very drowsy, and you should not feel pain during the procedure. It is generally a short process. Guided by ultrasound, the doctor passes a fine needle through the vaginal wall into each follicle and gently draws out the fluid. The eggs sit within that fluid and are passed straight to the embryology team, who begin working with them immediately.

You will need someone to take you home. Most people wake feeling groggy, slow or spaced out. You may notice cramping or bloating. You may feel emotional, relieved, overwhelmed or simply tired. It is common to want a blanket and a quiet place to rest. Some people feel proud of what their body has done. Others feel unexpectedly flat. There is no right emotional response here. You have just been through a lot.

Before you leave, or shortly after, you will be told how many eggs were collected.

Understanding egg numbers

Egg count is only one part of the story. People respond to stimulation in their own way, and the number collected varies widely. Age, ovarian reserve, medical history and the way in which your hormones respond to medication all play a role. Some bodies produce many eggs in a treatment cycle. Others produce only a few. Both routes can still lead to pregnancy, because the path forwards depends on what those eggs do next rather than the number alone. What matters most is not the number collected, but what happens next:

- How many eggs are mature.
- How many fertilise.
- How many embryos develop well enough for transfer or freezing.

> **Radical honesty: It is true that having more eggs can increase the likelihood of reaching a chromosomally normal embryo. Biology has a numbers element to it, and it would be misleading to pretend otherwise. More eggs can create more embryos, and more embryos can create more chances.**
>
> **But here is what numbers cannot tell. They cannot predict which egg will be the one that continues to grow. They cannot determine who will become a parent and who will not. Egg quality, age, sperm health, laboratory conditions and pure biological chance all play roles that no amount of effort or perfection can control.**

This is especially hard for those who are used to working hard and seeing results. The high achievers. The planners. The people who believe that if they pour everything in, the outcome should follow. IVF does not always reward effort in that linear way, which can feel deeply unfair.

A small number of strong eggs can matter far more than a large number that struggle to progress. One healthy embryo can be enough to change a life. Lower numbers are not a judgement on you or your body. They are one part of the picture, not the whole story.

If you leave the egg collection appointment with fewer eggs than you hoped for, it is human to feel sad, frustrated or shaken. You do not have to rush yourself into optimism. You are allowed to take a breath and let the feeling move through. In time, if you choose to continue, your team may adapt the stimulation, medication, timing or approach based on how your body responded. Each treatment cycle teaches something.

While your eggs are being collected, the focus also turns to sperm.

Stage three: sperm collection and preparation

For many people, sperm is provided on the same day as egg collection. This usually involves producing a sample through masturbation into a sterile pot in a private clinic room. The timing matters, because the embryology team aims to work with fresh sperm as soon as the eggs arrive in the laboratory.

You may hear people say that this is the male partner's 'one job', and in practical terms that can sound true; however, it overlooks how much pressure sits inside this moment. Being asked to perform on demand, in a medical setting, with emotions running high, can make arousal and ejaculation harder rather than easier. And as we know, anxiety does not help the nervous system relax.

Clinics usually advise how long to abstain from ejaculation beforehand (usually two to five days), as this can support sperm quality. If there is any concern about producing a sample on the day, it is important to raise it early. In some circumstances, a back-up sample can be frozen in advance, or additional support can be planned so that no one is relying on a single pressured moment.

If there are known difficulties with erection, ejaculation or performance anxiety, medicines such as sildenafil may be prescribed to help. The best time to talk about this is well before egg collection day.

Once the sperm sample is given, it moves to the laboratory. Embryologists examine it carefully, looking at how many sperm are present, how well they move, what proportion have a typical shape and whether the sample appears healthy overall. If support is needed, specific techniques can be used to select the strongest sperm for fertilisation.

With both eggs and sperm now in the care of the laboratory, the visible part of treatment pauses. For you, this can feel difficult as you are, in essence, handing everything over and waiting to hear what happens next. That is the heart of the next stage.

Stage four: fertilisation and the first laboratory days

Once your eggs have been collected, they move into a different part of the process. In the laboratory, they are examined, prepared and combined with sperm. Depending on your fertility plan, this usually happens in one of two ways:

- In conventional IVF (*see* pp. 178–80), eggs and sperm are placed together in culture (the nutrient-rich liquid used in the IVF laboratory to keep eggs, sperm and embryos supported while they are outside the body) so that fertilisation can occur without direct intervention.
- In ICSI (*see* pp. 184–85), an embryologist selects one sperm for each mature egg and injects it directly inside.

Fertilisation usually takes place over the next 16–20 hours.

In a laboratory, this is a well-established and highly practised procedure. For you, however, this may feel like one of the most delicate stretches of IVF. Up until now, most of the effort has been held in your body. You have stimulated, injected, attended appointments, tolerated discomfort and shown up again and again. Now, the work continues somewhere you cannot see.

We have witnessed many times a particular complexity of feelings in this moment. Relief sits alongside a strange emptiness. You may feel as though you have handed over something precious and are waiting outside a room you cannot enter.

Radical honesty: The hard work your body has done until now is suddenly in the hands of the laboratory team, and that shift in responsibility can feel both comforting and unsettling at the same time.

The first phone call and what happens next

Most clinics will call you the day after egg collection to share how many eggs have been fertilised. *Fertilised* means that a sperm has successfully entered an egg and the embryologist has confirmed, usually around 16–18 hours later, that both sets of genetic material are present and the process has begun. This is checked under the microscope and is the first sign that fertilisation has taken place. When this happens, the resulting structure, known as a zygote, begins dividing. Over the following days, if development continues, it may grow into an embryo.

The call itself may last only minutes, yet it can feel momentous. You might find yourself watching your phone, checking for signal, jumping when it rings. You may write down every word. You may feel hopeful, unsettled, disappointed, relieved or unsure how to feel at all. All of these are understandable responses.

If the number of fertilised eggs is lower than you hoped, panic or sadness may surface quickly. It can help to remember that quantity is only one part of the picture. A small number of embryos that continue to grow can matter far more than a large number that do not progress.

After fertilisation, the embryos are placed into an incubator and cared for in controlled laboratory conditions. The environment is carefully regulated to mimic the body, giving the embryos the conditions they need to continue dividing and growing.

After the initial call, you may receive updates at particular points rather than each day.

Day 3: cleavage stage

Around day three, embryos are often at the *cleavage stage*. At this stage, they are dividing into more cells but have not yet formed specialised structures. They remain microscopic, and each division is part of their earliest development.

Day 5 or 6: blastocyst stage

By day five, or sometimes day six, some embryos may reach the *blastocyst stage*, which is more advanced (*see* p. 164). Because blastocysts have developed further, the clinic is able to learn more about their potential. These are often the embryos selected for transfer or freezing.

Radical honesty: Not all embryos will reach the blastocyst stage. Some stop developing before then, and although this can be hard to hear, it is a normal part of the process. A day three embryo can still lead to a healthy pregnancy and baby. A blastocyst offers more information, but it is not a guarantee of outcome.

Once embryos begin to divide and some reach blastocyst stage, clinics will often assess them more closely. This process is known as embryo grading, and it helps guide planning for transfer or freezing.

Embryo grading

Embryo grading is a way of assessing how an embryo looks and behaves as it develops. It helps clinicians make informed decisions about which embryos may be suitable for transfer and which may be frozen for future use. Grading cannot predict the outcome with certainty, but it offers a helpful snapshot of how the embryo is progressing at this stage.

Most clinics use a similar approach to grading, although systems vary slightly. In general, the team looks at how the cells are dividing, how even they appear and how well the embryo is organising itself as it matures.

How embryos are graded

Embryos are usually checked at set points. The most common are day two or three, and then again on day five or six.

Day 2 to day 3: early cell division

At this stage, embryos are often between four and eight cells. Embryologists pay attention to the following aspects:

- How many cells are present.
- Whether the cells are similar in size.
- How evenly they are dividing.

An embryo that is developing well tends to divide steadily, with cells that look quite similar to each other. This does not guarantee success, but it suggests healthy early development.

Day 5 or day 6: blastocyst stage

By day five or six, some embryos reach the blastocyst stage. This is a more mature point where the embryo has organised into two parts:

- The inner cell mass (which may become the baby).
- The trophectoderm (which may form the placenta).

What grading is looking for

Grading focuses on a few main features:

- Cell number and symmetry: Embryos that have the expected number of cells for their stage and cells that are similar in size are often considered higher quality. This suggests steady development.
- Fragmentation: Sometimes, small pieces break off from cells. This is called fragmentation. A little fragmentation is common. A lot can indicate that the embryo may be under stress or struggling to develop smoothly. Even so, embryos with fragmentation have created babies.
- Blastocyst development: When grading blastocysts, embryologists look at how expanded the embryo is, how healthy the inner cell

mass appears and how cohesive the trophectoderm layer looks. Expansion helps the blastocyst prepare to hatch from its shell and implant in the uterus.

The Gardner system

You may come across letters or numbers during conversations with the embryologists. This is often the Gardner grading system, which is commonly used in the UK. You may see a number and two letters used to describe a blastocyst. The number relates to how expanded the blastocyst has become, while the letters describe the appearance of the inner cell mass and trophectoderm. In general, higher quality grades suggest that the embryo appears to be developing well, but grading can never predict with certainty whether an embryo will implant or result in a baby.

However, outcomes are never guaranteed either way.

It is more helpful to ask your clinic to explain what your specific grade means than to decode letters on your own.

Radical honesty: Some of the embryos that become babies are not the ones everyone expected. A lower-graded embryo can result in a healthy pregnancy, while a beautifully graded embryo may not implant. Grading offers guidance, not certainty.

Grading is like looking at a photograph taken at the very beginning of a journey. It shows what we can see today: the structure, the organisation, the early signs of growth. What it cannot do is tell the future. It simply helps your team decide where to place the next step.

Once grading is complete and decisions have been made about transfer or freezing, attention shifts back towards your body. The next part of the process is preparing the place where an embryo may be invited to settle.

Stage five: preparing the uterus and embryo transfer

You may hear your clinic talk about your 'lining' when preparing for embryo transfer. This refers to the uterine (or endometrial) lining, the tissue inside the uterus where an embryo would attach.

In IVF, a *good lining* is one that looks receptive. Thickness is one part of this, and most clinics hope to see around 7–8mm or more. Some prefer 9mm, and some people conceive with slightly thinner linings. Numbers are useful, but they are not absolute rules. Professor Mustafa Baris Ata and colleagues have also published research suggesting there may not be one exact lining measurement that determines success or failure. While clinics still look for reassuring signs of receptivity, pregnancies can and do occur with thinner linings.

Structure matters too. On ultrasound, many clinics look for a *trilaminar* or *triple line* appearance, which means the lining has a layered look that tends to be associated with readiness for implantation. Again, this is a guide rather than a guarantee.

A good lining is one that appears thick enough, well organised and well supplied with blood flow, creating a soft landing place for an embryo to settle.

Radical honesty: Lining measurements can cause a lot of anxiety. It is common to watch every millimetre and wonder if it is enough. Lining changes over days, and it can continue to improve right up to transfer. A single scan is not the whole story. Your clinic can adjust your medication if needed, and many linings that seem borderline at first grow into something suitable with time and support.

Progesterone support

As the lining develops, most IVF clinics introduce progesterone to support implantation (*see* pp. 222–24). In a natural menstrual cycle, progesterone rises after ovulation to prepare the uterine lining for a possible pregnancy. In IVF, that rhythm is often disrupted, especially after egg collection. Supplementing progesterone helps the lining remain receptive and supported until the placenta can take over.

Understanding progesterone levels

It is very normal for progesterone levels to rise and fall throughout the day. Levels vary depending on the type of progesterone you are using (*see* pp. 222–24), how your body absorbs it and when blood is taken. Small changes are expected and do not usually indicate a problem.

If levels fall significantly or remain low over time, your clinic may adjust the dose or change the route. Sometimes, this means increasing vaginal support. Sometimes, it means adding intramuscular injections, which can provide steadier levels in the bloodstream. The overall picture is more important than one isolated reading. If progesterone is consistently supported, it is likely doing what it needs to do.

Radical honesty: Progesterone support can bring hope and frustration in equal measure. Many people experience breast tenderness, bloating, fatigue or mood changes. These sensations can feel almost identical to early pregnancy, which makes the wait after transfer even more emotionally complex.

When the lining looks receptive and progesterone has been started, the focus moves towards the moment many people spend weeks anticipating: the transfer itself.

A word on how many embryos to transfer

Guidelines in the UK encourage single embryo transfer where possible. This is because twins or triplets carry higher risks for both parent and babies. In some situations, such as older age or lower-quality embryos, transferring two embryos may be discussed. It is usually a shared decision between you and your clinic, balancing hope with safety. The HFEA's patient guidance explicitly states that when a top-quality embryo (often a blastocyst) is available, best practice is to transfer only one embryo.

Radical honesty: The aim of treatment is not just a pregnancy. It is a healthy pregnancy.

In the spirit of radical honesty, in some circumstances patients may discuss transferring more than one embryo with their clinic. Decisions about the number of embryos to transfer are based on a range of factors, including age, embryo quality, a history of previous failed IVF attempts and/or pregnancy losses, and whether genetic testing (PGT-A) results are available. Where an embryo is known to be chromosomally normal, transferring a single embryo is usually recommended. Where genetic testing has not been carried out, transferring two embryos may be a reasonable option for some patients, depending on their history. It is never a straightforward decision, and should always involve a careful discussion with your fertility team about the potential benefits and risks, including those associated with multiple pregnancy.

The embryo transfer procedure

Embryo transfer is usually a gentle and relatively quick procedure carried out in a clinic room. Sedation is not usually needed, and you can often have a partner or support person with you.

The doctor or nurse will place a speculum into the vagina, as with a smear test, then pass a thin, flexible catheter through the cervix into the uterus. The embryo or embryos are loaded into this catheter in a tiny volume of fluid. With ultrasound guidance, the clinician gently releases the embryo into the uterine cavity.

Many people choose to watch the screen as this happens. Often, you will see a tiny, bright flash of fluid appear in the darker space of the uterus.

Some describe this as a sacred or surreal moment. For others, it feels calm and almost anticlimactic. You might cry, smile, squeeze a hand or simply feel tired and ready to go home.

Radical honesty: There can be a quiet pressure to feel that this moment is magical. You are in charge of how you want to feel in this moment.

After a brief rest, most people go home the same day. Physically, you can often return to normal gentle activity. Emotionally, you step into what many describe as the hardest part of treatment: the wait. That is where we go next.

Stage six: the two-week wait

Once an embryo has been transferred into the uterus, there is a waiting period of around two weeks before a pregnancy test can reliably be taken to see whether the transfer has been successful. This is commonly known as the 'two-week wait'. From this point, the frequency of appointments often reduces and instructions become lighter.

From the outside, life may seem to return to normal. Inside, it rarely feels that simple. For many people, the two-week wait is one of the most emotionally demanding phases of IVF. There is very little to do but wait, hold hope and move through uncertainty one day at a time.

You may become more aware of your body than ever before. Twinges, heaviness, cramping, bloating, tiredness, breast tenderness, changes in appetite or discharge and even spotting can all occur in this phase. Many of these sensations are influenced by progesterone and stimulation medications (*see* pp. 214–19), not necessarily by pregnancy itself. The body is busy and active, and symptoms can be misleading in both directions.

Radical honesty: Most people symptom-watch during the two-week wait. You may analyse every feeling, google late into the night, compare your experience with others or read forums or stories looking for clues. The truth is that medication can mimic pregnancy symptoms, and the absence of symptoms does not mean treatment has not worked. Your body cannot reliably tell you the outcome at this point.

Daily life in this phase

People cope with this wait in very different ways. Some continue life much as usual, keeping routines and work in place. Others slow down, take time off, prioritise rest or create softer days. Neither approach is right or wrong. You may find yourself moving between these states depending on mood, energy or how close test day feels.

Radical honesty: For the first two to three days, please take it easy. Rest when you can, keep life gentle and avoid pushing yourself. Short, relaxed walks are fine, but this is not the time for exertion, intense exercise or 'powering through'. Your body is doing important work. Giving it space to recover is part of the treatment.

It can help to keep a few thoughts close:

- You do not have to relax to make it work.
- You do not have to think positively to 'deserve' a pregnancy.
- Embryos need biology; you need care.

If you find yourself checking symptoms, counting days or scrolling online for reassurance, you are responding to uncertainty in a very natural way. You are trying to navigate hope and fear at the same time.

Spotting during the wait

Spotting/implantation bleeding refers to small amounts of bleeding, which are often noticeable only on wiping rather than requiring a pad. It may be pink, red or, most commonly, brown. Spotting can occur for a number of reasons, including progesterone irritation, cervical sensitivity after transfer or natural hormonal shifts. Spotting does not reliably indicate success or failure. Heavy bleeding should always be discussed with your clinic, but light spotting alone is common and does not automatically mean the treatment cycle has not worked.

CASE STUDY: DEBBIE, CHRIS AND THE TWO-WEEK WAIT

Debbie, 38, and her partner Chris, 40, had been trying to conceive for three years. After multiple failed attempts and a pregnancy loss, they decided to pursue IVF. Debbie's body responded well to stimulation, and a promising number of eggs were collected. They now found themselves in the waiting space after transfer.

Debbie was a primary school teacher who was known for her warmth and patience. During the two-week wait, she threw herself into work, staying late to plan lessons and organise school events. Teaching helped distract her, but the worry never fully left.

Midway through the wait, Debbie noticed spotting. Panic rose quickly, pulling painful memories of her pregnancy loss to the surface. Chris held her and tried to reassure her, but the fear lingered. Each cramp and twinge sent her mind racing.

Debbie began sleeping badly. At night, she scrolled through fertility forums and symptom-checking websites, hoping to find a story that matched her own and ended well. During the day, she held herself together for her pupils, but inside, she felt fragile and haunted by a sense of possible failure.

She and Chris had agreed not to test early. As the days passed, the test in the bathroom cabinet became harder to ignore. Part of her wanted to know as soon as possible to prepare. Part of her wanted to protect herself from finding out too soon.

Debbie's reactions were not a reflection of weakness or negativity. The two-week wait can make even the calmest and most rational people feel anxious, hypervigilant and emotionally overwhelmed. When so much matters, the mind naturally searches for certainty and protection wherever it can.

Debbie's experience is not unusual. Many people move through hope, fear, bargaining and resignation several times a day.

Radical honesty: The wait can feel cruel at times.

What happens next

Most clinics recommend testing around 10–14 days after transfer, using a blood test or a home pregnancy test depending on their protocol. The timing varies, but this moment is what the waiting builds towards.

Stage seven: pregnancy test day and what comes next

Test day. It may be tomorrow, next week or some time further ahead. Whenever it arrives, that day often carries more than a result alone. This day is not just about a line on a stick or a number in a result. It carries the weight of everything you have walked through so far: the injections, the appointments, the logistics, the waiting, the hope, the disappointment you may have survived before, the whispered conversations you had with yourself when nobody else could hear. It holds effort, longing and the possibility of a future imagined more than once.

The result you receive today may open a door, close one or leave you standing in the space between. However your outcome arrives, it deserves recognition, care and room to breathe.

There are three things that could possibly happen on this day.

If the result is negative

In our years working in fertility services, these were often the moments that stayed with us the longest. We walked beside many people right up to test day, holding hope with them. When the result was negative, we felt the weight of it too.

A negative test is not just the absence of pregnancy. It is the closing of a possibility you may have held deeply. It marks the end of a treatment cycle that carried your time, energy, money and hope. You may have imagined due dates, milestones, names or simply the feeling of holding the child you wanted so much. When that future falls away, grief is a natural response.

You might feel sad, angry, numb, flat, restless or unable to think clearly. You might want company or silence. You might want to plan again immediately or shut the door on treatment for now. Whatever you feel, it is allowed.

Radical honesty: This outcome is not your fault. You did not fail. You showed up for something difficult, and you hoped. That is courage, even if today it feels like loss.

What comes next

Most clinics offer a follow-up appointment to review the treatment cycle. These discussions can be helpful, but they can also feel raw. You are entitled to time and space, and you are entitled to ask questions. Decisions about trying again, pausing or considering other routes do not have to be made quickly.

Support can help here. Speaking to a therapist, joining a support group, talking with others who have walked a similar path or simply sharing how you feel with someone you trust can ease the isolation that often follows test day. You do not have to hold this alone.

If the result is unclear or equivocal

Sometimes, the answer is neither yes nor no. A faint line, a low human chorionic gonadotrophin (hCG) result or an hCG result that sits just below the expected range can place you in another wait. You may be asked to repeat blood tests after 48–72 hours, watching numbers rise, fall or hold. These days can feel suspended in time.

You might zoom in on test photos, analyse symptoms, compare numbers online and test again and again. You might move between hope and dread hour to hour. None of this means you are coping poorly. It means you care deeply about an outcome you cannot yet see clearly. Several paths are possible:

- Levels may rise and continue into a healthy pregnancy.
- They may rise slowly and remain uncertain for a time.
- They may fall, indicating the pregnancy is not continuing.
- Occasionally, further checks are needed to exclude ectopic pregnancy (*see* pp. 240–41).

Your clinic will guide you through these steps, though the wait can feel painfully slow.

> **Radical honesty: The grey zone can be one of the hardest emotional places. Hope without certainty and fear without closure ask a lot of you.**

If the result is positive

A positive result after IVF often lands with complexity. Joy, disbelief, relief, fear and quiet shock can sit together without cancelling one another out. You may stare at the test for far longer than seems necessary, waiting for it to prove itself. You may cry, laugh, sit in silence or feel strangely calm. All are natural responses to something momentous.

For many, early pregnancy after fertility treatment can feel delicate. You might check for spotting each time you go to the toilet. You may want to celebrate but find yourself holding back, protecting your heart until things feel more certain. This does not mean you are ungrateful. It means you remember what it took to get here.

> **Radical honesty: A positive result can bring happiness and fear side by side. It is possible to feel joy while still bracing for the unknown.**

Chapter 11 will walk with you through early pregnancy after treatment, including first scans, ongoing medication and the emotional landscape that follows. For now, it may be enough to know that cautious hope is a normal place to begin. And if you are reading this with a positive result, and it feels alright to receive it, we would love to offer you our congratulations.

Closing reflections

We have just worked our way through the seven key stages of IVF, from the first appointment to the day a pregnancy test gives its answer. You now know what happens inside your body., inside the clinic and inside the quiet emotional space that often sits between hope and uncertainty. If you are here, reading the final part of this chapter, we want to acknowledge what it takes to reach this point. IVF asks for time, money, planning, medication, patience, resilience and the willingness to try without knowing the outcome. That is not small; we think that is brave.

Some people will close this chapter with a positive result, and some will be carrying disappointment or loss. Others may be preparing to try again, or stepping back to breathe. These pages are for every person who has injected, waited, hoped, cried, googled at three in the morning or dared to imagine a future they cannot yet touch.

The road from here, sadly, divides. One path leads into early pregnancy and the chapter that follows. If you are walking that way, we will join you there, when you are ready, as you take your next steps.

The other path pauses here for now. If you are sitting in disappointment or waiting to gather strength before continuing, we see you. We are sorry. You have shown courage in getting this far. We hope with you that the door opens again ahead, and when it does, we will be here to support you.

Let's turn now to understanding what your options are and the different types of treatments you will meet along your way.

8

Types of fertility treatment

Before we begin, let's take a breath together.

If treatment is the next step for you, it is natural to arrive here holding more than one feeling at once. You might have sensed this was where things were heading while also wishing there had been another way. It is a complicated emotional space to stand in, and nothing about reaching this point is simple, but you do not have to move through the journey ahead alone. From here, we will guide you gently, helping you understand what lies ahead so it feels a little less overwhelming.

It can help to think of fertility treatment not as one big decision but as a series of smaller decisions that unfold gradually. Each stage brings new information: how your body responds, how your hormones behave, what the scans reveal and how you actually feel as you go through it. These insights shape the next steps. Treatment is not something you choose once and stay fixed to; it adapts with you.

In the early stages, many people have several possible pathways. As investigations progress, some options become more relevant, and others naturally fall away. This is how clarity builds in fertility care. But it can feel mentally heavy, because this journey is not only biological. It sits within a wider reality that includes NHS criteria, private choices, waiting lists, geography, finances, timing and the emotional support you have around you.

This is why two people with similar diagnoses may still be offered different routes. Your individual circumstances matter.

As you move forwards, you may also notice that treatment is far more flexible than it first appears. There will be moments when pausing feels right, and others when moving ahead is the only thing that feels bearable. There will be options that make sense for your stage of life, and others that simply don't. Allowing space for that flexibility often makes the whole process feel more manageable.

In this chapter, we will walk through the main treatment options most people in the UK are likely to encounter. We will start with the approaches that tend to come earlier in the pathway (ovulation induction and IUI) and then move on to treatments that bring more of the process into the clinic: IVF, frozen embryo transfer cycles and ICSI. From there, we will explore donor options, solo parenting, surrogacy, adoption and fertility preservation. Chapter 9 will then explore advanced testing and add-ons, which are often offered alongside treatment.

Before we begin, it is important to say that not every treatment is suitable for every person. This has nothing to do with failure or blame; it is about biology. For example:

- Ovulation induction will not help if you are already ovulating regularly.
- IUI is unlikely to work if your fallopian tubes are blocked.
- IVF may be recommended sooner if time is important (for example, if your ovarian reserve is low or age is a factor).
- Donor eggs or sperm may be the safest or most effective option when egg or sperm quality is significantly affected.

How to read this chapter

We are going to walk through the treatments in the following order:

- Ovulation induction
- Intrauterine insemination (IUI)
- In vitro fertilisation (IVF)
- Frozen embryo transfer (FET) cycles
- Intracytoplasmic sperm injection (ICSI)

And then we will move on to the following topics:

- Egg freezing and fertility preservation
- Donor eggs and sperm (including solo parenting)
- Surrogacy
- Adoption

At each step, we will explain what the treatment is, what it usually looks like in real life and where a radically honest perspective may help you approach it with more clarity and confidence.

Let's begin.

Ovulation induction: helping your body release an egg

Ovulation induction is often suggested as a first step when your body is not releasing eggs regularly, or at all. This treatment uses medication to encourage the ovaries to mature and release one egg, or sometimes two, to increase the chance of conception through intercourse or IUI (*see* pp. 177–78). Typically, ovulation induction involves the use of oral medications that stimulate the release of the hormones necessary for follicle development and ovulation. All of the medications you will come across are explained in chapter 10.

Ovulation induction is commonly used for people with irregular menstrual cycles, suspected ovulation problems or conditions such as PMOS (*see* pp. 30–31). It is usually one of the simplest and least-invasive treatments available.

What this looks like in real life

You will usually take tablets at home for a set number of days early in your menstrual cycle. Sometimes, injections are used, particularly if the tablets do not lead to ovulation. You may:

- Attend one or more ultrasound scans to check how many follicles are growing.
- Have blood tests to confirm hormone levels.
- Be asked to time intercourse or come in for IUI at the right point in your menstrual cycle.

You may hardly notice any changes, or you may experience hormonal side effects such as mood swings, headaches, breast tenderness or feeling more emotionally sensitive. There are usually no theatre procedures and no need for sedation.

Monitoring varies. Some NHS pathways offer minimal or no ultrasound monitoring, while many private clinics monitor more closely.

Less monitoring can make timing feel more uncertain. More monitoring can make life feel more medical.

> **Radical honesty: Ovulation induction can be a helpful first step and, for some people, it is all that is needed. For others, especially where time is already an issue, staying too long on ovulation induction can quietly cost precious months or even years. If you are in your mid-30s or older, if your ovarian reserve is low or if you have already been trying for a long time, it is worth asking your clinical team directly: 'If this does not work within a few treatment cycles, what is our next step, and when will we move to it?'**

CASE STUDY: RACHEL AND FABIO – STAYING ON ONE TREATMENT TOO LONG

Rachel, 35, had mild PMOS. Fabio's sperm test was normal. They were offered ovulation induction as a first step, and this made sense. It felt gentle and manageable.

After three unsuccessful treatment cycles, the medication was changed and the monitoring became more intensive. Another three cycles came and went. Each one carried its own build-up of hope and its own quiet collapse.

By the time they moved on to IVF, Rachel was 36. Her ovarian reserve had fallen since starting treatment. Fewer eggs were collected than might have been possible a year earlier.

Rachel and Fabio later said they wished someone had spoken with them more clearly about time. Ovulation induction had not been wrong. It had simply gone on for too long.

Rachel and Fabio's story (*see* above) shows how easy it is to stay with one approach while hoping it will eventually work, and how helpful it can be to pause and reconsider the direction of travel. For some people, the next step after ovulation induction is IUI, which offers a different rhythm and focus.

Intrauterine insemination (IUI)

IUI involves placing prepared sperm directly into the uterus close to the time of ovulation. It aims to help more sperm reach the egg by bypassing the cervix and shortening the distance they need to travel.

IUI may be used when there are mild sperm issues, unexplained infertility or situations where timing intercourse is difficult. It is also commonly used by same-sex female couples and solo parents using donor sperm.

What this looks like in real life

An IUI cycle often includes the following steps:

- Oral medication or, occasionally, injections to stimulate one or two follicles.
- One to three monitoring scans, depending on the clinic.
- Close tracking of ovulation through scans, blood tests or home ovulation tests.
- A short procedure where sperm are placed into the uterus via a thin catheter.

The procedure itself usually takes just a few minutes. Many people describe it as similar to a smear test. You can usually return to normal activity the same day.

However, emotionally, it can carry a lot of weight for something that feels quite simple on the surface. There is often a sense of *Did that work?* almost immediately. Then the two-week wait (*see* pp. 168–69) begins, and many people find that their thoughts repeatedly circle back to the question of whether this treatment cycle will be different.

> **Radical honesty: IUI can be a meaningful treatment, particularly when there is a clear reason to use it, such as donor sperm or mild sperm issues. However, in situations where the sperm are normal, the fallopian tubes are open and age is a concern, repeated IUI cycles can act as more of a delay than a bridge.**

IUI sits early in the treatment pathway and can be helpful in certain situations. When it is not likely to work or when you need more detailed information about your eggs, sperm or embryos, IVF is usually the next step your team will explore with you.

In vitro fertilisation (IVF)

IVF involves stimulating the ovaries to produce multiple eggs, retrieving them under sedation, fertilising them with sperm in the lab, growing embryos and then transferring one or more embryo back into the uterus.

It is often recommended in the following circumstances:

- When other treatments have not worked.
- When the fallopian tubes are blocked (*see* p. 40).
- In cases of moderate to severe male factor infertility (*see* chapter 4).
- In some cases of endometriosis (*see* pp. 36–39).
- When genetic testing of embryos is needed (*see* pp. 203–6).
- When time or ovarian reserve (*see* p. 35) are important factors.

What this looks like in real life

Life during an IVF cycle often feels structured and busy. You may do some or all of the following:

- Attend scans and blood tests every few days during stimulation.
- Give yourself daily injections at home for 10–14 days.
- Juggle work and life around early appointments and blood tests.
- Experience bloating, pelvic discomfort, mood changes, fatigue or tearfulness.
- Feel as if you are living in two parallel worlds: everyday life and treatment life.

Egg collection is done under sedation. This is usually a day that carries significant emotional weight. For many people, it represents a turning point: the moment when weeks or months of injections, hope and uncertainty are distilled into a single outcome. It is the first time you are told how many eggs have been collected and, sometimes, whether any have been retrieved. For some, this brings relief or validation; for others, it can be confronting or disappointing. Either way, it is the point at which effort and emotion become tangible and where possibility begins to feel more real.

After fertilisation, you are often updated on how many eggs were fertilised and how many embryos continue to grow. Embryo transfer usually happens a few days later. It is often a gentler procedure, usually without sedation.

Radical honesty: IVF is not simply a medical protocol. It is a psychological and relational experience. It demands time, energy, logistical planning, financial decision-making and emotional resilience.

IVF can significantly increase the chance of pregnancy when other treatments have not worked, but it cannot override biology entirely. A strong treatment cycle may result in multiple embryos for future use, while a weaker cycle can still offer valuable information about how your eggs respond and how fertilisation unfolds in the laboratory.

Our advice is to try to think of it like this: success in IVF is not measured only in terms of pregnancy. It also lies in the clarity it can bring and the next steps it can help you define. IVF can give you information, create options, provide embryos to freeze for the future and offer a clearer understanding of how your body responds within the limits of what medicine can currently do.

Once embryos have been created through IVF, there are two main approaches to embryo transfer depending on timing. In some cases, an embryo is transferred within the same treatment cycle, a process known as 'fresh' (or traditional) embryo transfer. In others, embryos are frozen and transferred in a later cycle; this is called frozen embryo transfer (FET). Both approaches fall fully within IVF; the difference lies not in how embryos are created but in when they are transferred into the uterus. We will discuss FET in more detail below.

Frozen embryo transfer (FET) cycles

In recent years, FET has become a common approach in the UK. Many clinics now favour transferring embryos in a later treatment cycle after freezing and thawing them, rather than immediately after retrieval. This change reflects a broader trend in IVF practice: a move away from routine fresh transfers more towards prioritising safety, individualised timing and optimised conditions for implantation. Here are the reasons why they are now more common:

Greater use of genetic testing

More patients are choosing to test embryos, with the increased use of preimplantation genetic testing for aneuploidy (PGT-A). Aneuploidy refers to an abnormal number of chromosomes in an embryo, while a euploid embryo has the correct number of chromosomes and is therefore more likely to result in a healthy pregnancy (*see* p. 205). Because the results take time, embryos are usually frozen while the report is processed. A frozen cycle then allows transfer when the information is clear and timing can be planned.

Improved freezing techniques

Modern freezing techniques (known as vitrification) have transformed outcomes. Embryos now survive thawing at very high rates, making frozen transfer a reliable option that was not possible in the early days of IVF.

Potential benefits for specific groups

Some clinics report similar or better outcomes with FET in situations such as:

- High ovarian response.
- Risk of ovarian hyperstimulation syndrome (OHSS; *see* p. 157).
- Raised progesterone levels at trigger (*see* p. 218).
- The need for immune or uterine lining preparation (*see* p. 202).
- When PGT-tested embryos are used (*see* pp. 203–6).

This does not apply to everyone, but it highlights why frozen cycles are often considered.

More control and flexibility

With a frozen cycle, there is time to prepare the uterine lining, balance hormones and support the immune environment, if relevant. This can help the transfer feel calmer, more paced and less bound to the timing of stimulation.

Safety

In those at risk of OHSS, skipping a fresh transfer can reduce complications. FET is often chosen for this reason alone.

Types of FET cycle

At this stage of treatment, the embryos have already been created. The focus now shifts to preparing the uterus for the embryo transfer. There are two main ways in which this can be done.

A natural frozen cycle

A natural frozen cycle works with your own hormones rather than replacing them. The aim is to identify the moment when your body naturally prepares for implantation and to transfer the embryo at that point.

You will usually attend a small number of scans to follow your developing follicle and monitor the lining of your uterus. Your clinic may also use blood tests to check your oestrogen and progesterone levels, or to confirm ovulation. Once your team can see that you are about to ovulate, they will plan the transfer for the appropriate day, matching the natural window in which an embryo would normally arrive in the uterus.

This approach can feel appealing if your menstrual cycles are regular and predictable. It often involves fewer medications and fewer appointments, which can help the process feel more manageable. Some people appreciate the sense that their body is taking the lead, with the clinic stepping in only at the key moment.

However, a natural cycle is not always suitable, especially if your menstrual cycles vary each month or if the unpredictability of monitoring ovulation feels difficult to manage. In these situations, a medicated frozen cycle may offer more stability and clearer planning.

A medicated frozen cycle

A medicated frozen cycle uses prescribed hormones to prepare the lining of your uterus in a steady and controlled way. Oestrogen is administered first, usually as tablets, patches or, occasionally, gel. This encourages the lining to grow to the thickness needed for implantation. You will have one or more scans to check how the lining is developing. When it reaches the desired pattern and thickness, progesterone is introduced.

Progesterone is the hormone that transforms the uterine lining from a growing environment to a receptive one. The timing of progesterone is crucial, as the embryo is transferred only after a set number of hours or days of progesterone exposure. Because everything is controlled hormonally, your clinic can schedule the transfer precisely, which many people find reassuring.

A medicated cycle can be helpful if your menstrual cycles are irregular, if ovulation is unpredictable or if your clinic has seen that you respond better when the environment is created rather than relied upon naturally. It can also make the process easier if you are working, travelling or juggling responsibilities, as timing becomes more planned.

Some people find the medications straightforward, while others notice side effects such as bloating, breast tenderness, mood shifts or fatigue. This is normal, and your clinic should explain what to expect.

Both approaches aim to create the same thing: a stable, receptive environment for an embryo.

Why might FET cycles perform as well as or better than fresh IVF cycles?

- In a frozen cycle, the body is not recovering from stimulation.
- The uterine lining can be prepared more deliberately and gently.
- The hormonal environment may be more physiologically stable, especially for those who had a strong response in their IVF cycle.

That said, the outcome still depends on the same core factors in both fresh and frozen transfers:

- Embryo quality.
- Your age at egg collection.
- How well your lining responds in the frozen cycle.
- Underlying medical or uterine factors.

One reassuring aspect of frozen cycles is that each embryo represents another opportunity. You do not need to repeat stimulation or egg collection, and for many people, success arrives through a frozen transfer rather than the first fresh one.

The emotional pace

Frozen cycles often feel quieter and more spacious than fresh cycles. You may find you can continue daily life more easily due to not having your ovaries stimulated with daily injections and fewer appointments being required for this approach to treatment. Many people describe frozen cycles as less overwhelming, although the emotional investment is still significant: waiting to see whether an embryo will implant carries its own weight, even in a calmer cycle.

For some people, a frozen transfer brings the outcome they have been hoping for. For others, the process highlights that they may need more information about fertilisation itself.

When implantation does not occur despite good-quality embryos and a carefully prepared uterine lining, clinicians look back at earlier stages of the IVF process to see whether fertilisation itself could be contributing. This is where ICSI may be discussed. ICSI is a form of IVF where an embryologist injects the sperm into the egg using a microscope instead of allowing natural selection to take place.

Intracytoplasmic sperm injection (ICSI)

ICSI is a technique used within IVF where an embryologist injects a single sperm directly into each mature egg. The rest of the process is the same as IVF. It is commonly used when the following circumstances apply:

- Sperm counts are very low.
- Sperm movement or shape is significantly affected.
- There has been failed fertilisation in a previous IVF cycle.
- Surgical sperm retrieval (*see* pp. 97–98) has been needed.

For many people, ICSI brings a sense of reassurance, as one more barrier has been intentionally removed.

> **Radical honesty: ICSI has transformed the treatment of male factor infertility (*see* chapter 4). Even when sperm numbers are extremely low or movement or shape are affected, fertilisation can still happen successfully. The embryologist selects a single healthy sperm and places it directly into the egg, which bypasses the need for the sperm to swim to or penetrate the egg on its own. For many couples, only a very small number of sperm are needed for ICSI to work. This can offer real hope, even when the semen analysis looks challenging.**

However, ICSI is not necessary for everyone. It does not increase the overall chance of pregnancy compared with standard IVF unless there is a clear sperm-related reason for using it. Its purpose is not to make IVF 'more successful' but to prevent fertilisation problems when sperm cannot fertilise the egg reliably on their own.

Using ICSI routinely when sperm are normal is unlikely to improve outcomes and adds cost. You are entitled to ask, 'Is there a specific reason you recommend ICSI in my case?'

ICSI completes the group of treatments that focus on bringing eggs and sperm together in the most supported way possible. From here, the pathway widens again. Not every family is built through partnered treatment, and many people choose to pursue parenthood in different and equally meaningful ways. They may not be ready to begin treatment, or they may want to keep open the possibility of having a biological child in the future. This is where fertility preservation comes in. Fertility preservation offers time, flexibility and a sense of choice at moments when life circumstances, medical conditions or age-related changes make the future feel uncertain. Let's explore what that looks like.

Egg freezing and fertility preservation

Fertility preservation is a way of storing eggs, sperm or embryos so that they can be used in the future. It can offer a sense of choice and stability at moments when time, health or circumstance may otherwise limit your options. Preservation is not only about medical technique. It is also about creating space to think, plan and move forwards without feeling rushed.

Who considers fertility preservation?

People freeze eggs, sperm or embryos for many reasons:

- They are not ready to try for a baby but want to protect their future fertility.
- They are having treatment for cancer or other medical conditions that may affect their fertility.
- They have a low ovarian reserve and want to store eggs while they still can.
- They are transitioning gender and want to have biological options later.
- They are in a relationship but not yet ready to conceive.
- They are beginning IVF and want to freeze embryos for later use.

There is no single story of who chooses preservation. It is a flexible, future-orientated decision that can support a wide range of life paths.

Egg freezing

Egg freezing involves stimulating the ovaries to grow multiple eggs, which are then retrieved through a short procedure and frozen using a rapid freezing technique called vitrification. The quality and quantity of the eggs depend largely on age and ovarian reserve. Freezing eggs in your early 30s typically offers higher success rates than freezing them later, but meaningful benefit is still possible for many people in their mid-30s.

Egg freezing does not guarantee a future pregnancy, but it can create a safety net that may ease some of the pressure many people feel as they navigate work, relationships and ageing.

> **Radical honesty: Egg freezing can be a valuable option for preserving fertility, but it is not an insurance policy or guarantee of a future baby. In general, embryos tend to survive the freezing and thawing process more reliably than unfertilised eggs, which is why embryo freezing usually has higher success rates overall. The age eggs are frozen at, the number collected and future sperm quality all still matter. Egg freezing preserves possibility, not certainty.**

Sperm freezing

Sperm freezing is straightforward. It involves producing a sperm sample that is then processed and frozen in small batches. Sperm can remain viable for many years. Sperm freezing can be especially important for people undergoing cancer treatment, taking medications that affect fertility or beginning gender-affirming hormones. It is also an option for anyone who would like to preserve fertility for the future.

Embryo freezing

Embryo freezing is different from egg or sperm freezing because it requires both eggs and sperm at the time of freezing. Embryos are created through IVF, grown for several days in the laboratory and then frozen. Frozen embryos often survive thawing very well (*see* p. 181). This option is commonly used by couples planning to delay pregnancy or by people who want the reassurance of embryos that are stored safely before moving into later stages of life.

Medical fertility preservation

The NHS provides fertility preservation for people whose medical treatment may affect fertility. This includes chemotherapy, radiotherapy, some surgeries and certain long-term medications. If this applies to you, your oncology or medical team should discuss this early so that preservation can happen before treatment begins.

Storage and legal considerations

In the UK, eggs, sperm and embryos can usually be stored for up to 55 years, provided consent forms are renewed at set intervals. Your clinic will guide you through this process. It is important to keep your contact details up to date, as storage regulations require ongoing consent.

Donor eggs and donor sperm

When we talk about a donor in fertility treatment, we mean a person who chooses to allow the use of their eggs or sperm, either as a known donor (donating to a family member or friend, for example) or as a donor through a licensed clinic or egg or sperm bank. Using a donor does not always mean using both donor eggs and donor sperm. In many cases, only one donor is involved, while the other element comes from the intended parent or their partner.

Donor eggs or sperm may be recommended in the following scenarios:

- Egg or sperm quality is severely reduced or sperm are absent.
- There is a high risk of passing on a serious genetic condition.
- Previous treatment cycles with your own eggs or sperm have repeatedly been unsuccessful.
- You are a same-sex couple or a solo parent using donor sperm or donor eggs.

You may see or hear the word 'gamete' at this stage, which refers to reproductive cells. Eggs and sperm are both gametes. Donor conception means using donor gametes to create embryos.

Solo parenting

Solo parenting through fertility treatment is an increasingly common and valid path to family building. It may be considered in a number of circumstances:

- You are single and feel ready to become a parent.
- You do not want to wait any longer to find a partner.
- There is a medical reason to act sooner, such as reduced ovarian reserve or planned cancer treatment.

Solo parenthood can take different forms depending on the biology involved. Some people pursue IVF or IUI with donor sperm. In other situations, intended parents may build their family through the use of donor eggs and a gestational surrogate. Although the pathways differ, the central theme is the same: choosing to create a family as one parent rather than within a partnership. You may need to take the following steps:

- Think about financial planning for both treatment and future parenting.
- Build a support network that will help with practical and emotional needs.
- Reflect on how you will talk to your child in the future about their conception story and family structure.

Some people who choose a solo path build their family with their own eggs or sperm. Others reach a moment when using their own eggs or sperm is no longer possible or advisable, and donor eggs or donor sperm become part of the conversation. Donor treatment is not only a medical option. It is also an emotional and relational decision, and it deserves time, clarity and compassion.

> **Radical honesty: Solo parenting is not second-best. It is a deliberate choice to create a family in a different way. Many people feel proud of that decision, even if it comes with moments of loneliness or worry.**

What information will you see about a donor?

The level of information you receive varies depending on the source of the donor eggs or sperm and the country of origin. UK donor profiles usually include physical characteristics such as height, hair and eye colour, ethnicity and, sometimes, a short personal statement or staff impressions.

International sperm banks may offer more extensive profiles. Some provide personality questionnaires, audio interviews, written essays, baby photos or childhood photos. In some countries, particularly the United States, adult photos may be available if the donor has consented to that level of openness. These differences can create the impression of 'levels', but they relate to donor consent and cultural norms rather than quality.

> **RIGHTS OF DONOR-CONCEIVED CHILDREN**
>
> In the UK, donors are identifiable to donor-conceived children once they turn 18. This means that while you will receive only non-identifying information at the time you choose your donor, your future child will have the legal right to request identifying details when they are an adult. Many people find this reassuring. For others, it raises questions about future conversations and identity. Your clinic and specialist counsellors can help you navigate this thoughtfully.

How it works

Donor sperm

If you are using donor sperm, your treatment may involve IUI or IVF depending on your medical situation, your age, and what your clinic feels is most likely to give you the best chance. Donor sperm is sourced from a licensed sperm bank, either in the UK or internationally, and every donor must meet strict screening requirements. These include testing for infectious diseases, a detailed family medical history, genetic conditions and lifestyle factors.

Types of donor sperm

You may notice terms such as these:

- IUI-prepared sperm
- IVF-prepared sperm
- Washed or unwashed sperm

These terms describe how the sample has been processed, not the suitability or quality of the donor. IUI requires sperm to be washed and prepared in a way that removes seminal fluid and concentrates the healthiest sperm. IVF-prepared sperm is processed differently because it will be used in the laboratory rather than placed directly into the uterus. Some clinics will ask whether the sample is washed or unwashed because they need a specific preparation for the type of treatment being carried out.

How donor sperm is used in treatment

If you are having IUI, the prepared sperm are placed directly into your uterus at the right moment in your menstrual cycle. This may be a natural or a medicated cycle, depending on your circumstances and your clinic's recommendation.

If IVF is recommended (*see* pp. 178–80), the donor sperm is used to fertilise your eggs in the laboratory. The resulting embryos can then be transferred fresh or frozen for future treatment cycles. In some cases, your clinic may suggest using ICSI (*see* pp. 184–85) with donor sperm, particularly if your eggs require a more precise fertilisation method.

Donor eggs

Using donor eggs is an option when your own eggs are unlikely to lead to a healthy pregnancy, or when treatment would carry risks that make donor eggs the safer choice. This may be due to age-related changes in egg quality, diminished ovarian reserve, previous IVF outcomes, early menopause, genetic conditions or certain medical histories. Some people arrive at donor eggs after many treatments, and others consider it early on.

Donor eggs can offer a significant increase in success rates, because the eggs usually come from younger donors who have undergone thorough screening. In the UK, all donors must meet strict medical, genetic and lifestyle criteria to ensure their eggs are suitable for treatment. Donor eggs may also be used in surrogacy arrangements, including for male couples or single men who are building their family through gestational surrogacy (*see* pp. 191–94).

Where donor eggs come from

Most people in the UK use eggs from the sources listed below:

- Anonymous identifiable UK donors recruited through clinics.
- Imported donor eggs from EU or US donor banks.
- A known donor, such as a sister, friend or relative.

How treatment works

Using donor eggs always involves IVF or ICSI because the eggs need to be fertilised before being transferred. If you will be carrying the pregnancy yourself, the process typically looks like this:

- The donor undergoes ovarian stimulation and egg collection.
- The eggs are fertilised with either your partner's sperm or donor sperm.
- The embryos grow in the laboratory.
- One or more embryo is transferred to your uterus in either a fresh or a frozen cycle.

If you are using frozen donor eggs, you will be involved in the fertilisation and transfer stages only. The donor's part took place before the eggs were frozen.

You will usually prepare your uterine lining with oestrogen and progesterone for a planned FET cycle, which allows your clinic to schedule treatment precisely.

Emotional considerations

Arriving at donor eggs or donor sperm can feel like a crossroads. You may feel relief that there is still a path forward. You may feel grief, sadness or a deep sense of ambivalence. All of these reactions are normal, and none of them mean you are making the wrong decision. There is no single emotional script for this part of the journey. Many people discover that their idea of family becomes clearer over time, not in a single moment of certainty.

Choosing a donor is not purely a medical decision. It often stirs emotions you may not have anticipated. You may notice moments of hope, curiosity, uncertainty, grief or protectiveness. All of these are understandable. Donor conception touches identity, family stories and the future conversations you may one day have with your child.

It can also help to remember that genetics is only one strand in the experience of becoming a parent. Bonding, love, caregiving, attunement and the story you build with your child are shaped through relationship, not DNA. This understanding does not erase loss, but it can make room for the family you are creating. As healthcare professionals, we have cared for many patients who took this road, with great results.

In the UK, counselling is formally recommended – and in some situations required – for anyone considering donor eggs and sperm. Beyond regulatory compliance, it is often deeply supportive. It provides space to explore emotions, values, what feels important to you in a donor and long-term implications. The latter include how donor conception may be spoken about within your family over time, how you feel about genetic difference within your family and how you might talk to your future child about their conception. It helps you think through what matters to you and approach this path with steadiness and intention.

Some people using donor eggs go on to carry the pregnancy themselves. Others reach a point where carrying a pregnancy is not possible or not safe. In other situations, such as for male couples or single men building their family, a gestational surrogate is part of the pathway from the beginning. When that happens, surrogacy becomes an important part of the conversation.

Surrogacy

Surrogacy becomes part of the conversation when the main barrier to pregnancy is not egg quality or sperm quality but the ability to carry a pregnancy safely. This may be due to medical conditions affecting the uterus, repeated pregnancy loss, a history of complex treatment, early menopause or circumstances such as being a same-sex male couple or a single man. Surrogacy is not a last resort. It is a meaningful and intentional way to build a family when biology or health creates limits that cannot be overcome safely.

In the UK, surrogacy is legal, but it operates within a specific legal framework that prioritises the welfare of the child, the surrogate and the intended parents. It is also an emotionally complex pathway that requires time, clarity and support.

Types of surrogacy

There are two forms of surrogacy:

- Traditional surrogacy: The surrogate's own egg is used, making her the genetic parent. This can be done through insemination with sperm from the intended father or a donor. Traditional surrogacy is less common in the UK because it brings additional emotional and legal complexity.
- Gestational surrogacy: An embryo is created through IVF using either the intended mother's egg or a donor egg and sperm from either the intended father or a donor. The surrogate carries the pregnancy but has no genetic link to the child. This is the most common form of surrogacy in the UK and is generally the preferred route.

WHERE TO FIND A SURROGATE

Most surrogacy in the UK happens through one of these routes:

- UK surrogacy organisations
- Independent matching through social networks
- International surrogacy agencies (although the legal frameworks vary significantly)

The treatment process

Surrogacy always involves IVF or ICSI because an embryo must be created before transfer. The usual steps are as follows:

- Embryos are created using your eggs or donor eggs.
- The eggs are fertilised with your partner's sperm or donor sperm.
- Either the embryos are frozen or you proceed with a fresh transfer.
- The surrogate's uterus is prepared with a medicated cycle.
- The embryo is transferred into the surrogate.
- The surrogate is supported through pregnancy and birth.

Clinics assess both the intended parents and the surrogate to ensure everyone is medically and emotionally prepared. Counselling is mandatory and usually very helpful.

Legal considerations

This is often the most confusing part for intended parents, so clarity matters:

- Under UK law, the surrogate is the legal mother at birth, regardless of genetics.
- If she is married or in a civil partnership, her spouse is the second legal parent unless they formally opt out.
- The intended parents must apply for a parental order after the birth to become the child's legal parents.

This process can feel counterintuitive for people who are genetically related to the baby, but it is the mechanism the law uses to safeguard everyone involved. Most surrogates and intended parents describe this stage as administrative rather than adversarial.

International surrogacy creates additional layers, including citizenship, passports and dual legal recognition. Specialist legal advice is essential.

The UK operates under an altruistic model. Surrogates cannot be paid beyond reasonable expenses. Overseas arrangements may involve compensated surrogacy, which is legal abroad but requires careful legal planning for intended parents returning to the UK.

Surrogacy frameworks vary widely from country to country. Some nations have excellent regulation, strong legal protections and clear ethical guidelines. Others may lack robust oversight or operate in ways that put surrogates, children or intended parents at risk. It is crucial to research carefully, work with reputable clinics and agencies only and, if pursuing an overseas arrangement, consult a UK fertility law specialist before making any commitments.

Emotional experience

Surrogacy offers hope where other treatments cannot, but it can also bring up layered feelings. Many people describe moments of:

- Relief that there is still a path to parenthood.
- Grief about not carrying the pregnancy.
- Deep gratitude towards the surrogate.
- Fear of things beyond their control.
- Protectiveness and uncertainty.

These feelings are understandable and do not mean you are ambivalent about becoming a parent. Surrogacy asks you to imagine a different version of family building from the one you may have pictured earlier in your life. It is normal for this to take time.

Surrogates themselves also navigate a complex emotional process. Good communication, honesty and thoughtful matching help everyone feel safe and supported.

Radical honesty: Surrogacy asks you to trust others in ways that can feel vulnerable. It also requires patience, flexibility and a willingness to share parts of your story with another person who is helping you build your family.

For many people, surrogacy becomes a story not of limitation but of collaboration, generosity and deep intention, as it is one way to build a family when pregnancy is not possible or not safe. Another path, which is equally meaningful and often misunderstood, is adoption.

Adoption

Adoption offers a route to parenthood that does not rely on pregnancy or genetics. It is a way of creating a family by giving a child a permanent, stable and loving home. In the UK, adoption is regulated, thorough and child-centred. The process is designed to ensure that the needs of the child, the birth family and the adoptive parents are carefully considered and supported. While it can feel long or emotionally exposing, the intention is to create the best possible match for everyone involved.

Who can adopt

Adoption in the UK is open to all of the following:

- Single parents
- Couples in long-term relationships
- LGBTQ+ parents
- People with or without children
- Individuals across a wide range of ages

You do not have to own a home, have a particular income or be in perfect circumstances to adopt. What matters is your capacity to offer safety, stability and emotional availability.

The assessment process

The adoption process usually involves a number of steps:

- An initial enquiry.
- Preparation workshops.
- Background checks and medical assessments.
- Several months of home study.
- Approval from an adoption panel.
- Matching with a child.
- A period of introductions.
- Placement.
- A legal adoption order.

The process is detailed by design. It helps you understand trauma, attachment, identity and how to meet the needs of a child who may have experienced loss or early adversity.

Children who need adoption

Most children in the UK who need adoption have experienced disruption in their early relationships. Some have been removed from their birth families for reasons related to safety. Others have been cared for by multiple people in their first years of life.

Adoption is not only about providing a home. It is about becoming a healing relationship for a child whose early story may include pain, confusion or neglect. This does not make adoption less joyful. It simply means the child's emotional world forms a core part of the process.

SUPPORT FOR ADOPTIVE FAMILIES

Adoptive families can access ongoing support through their agency, local authorities, therapists who specialise in adoption and trauma and organisations such as Adoption UK. Requesting support is not a sign of difficulty. It is a normal part of building secure attachments after a child has experienced early loss.

Adoption does not replace the path you hoped for. It becomes its own path. And for many people, it becomes the one that feels most aligned with who they are and the kind of family they want to create.

While adoption offers a way to build a family without pregnancy or genetics, some people reach a different point in their journey. The next chapter gets even more complex as we look more closely at advanced testing and add-ons, which are often offered alongside treatment. Understanding what they are, what they can and cannot tell you and when they may genuinely help can make it easier to navigate recommendations without feeling overwhelmed or pressured.

9

Advanced testing and add-ons

Few areas of fertility treatment generate as much discussion and differing opinion as advanced testing and add-ons. Some clinicians see certain technologies as exciting progress and important personalised care. Others worry that parts of the field are moving faster than the evidence. The reality often sits somewhere in between. Some parts of fertility care are considered core. Blood tests, ultrasound scans, stimulation medication, egg collection and embryo transfer usually sit in this category, as we discussed in chapter 8. These are the steps most people expect when they think about treatment. Alongside these, you may be offered further procedures or tests. These are sometimes called 'add-ons', and they include investigations that look more closely at the lining of the uterus, the microbiome, the immune system, the fallopian tubes and the genetic health of embryos. Some of these procedures are well established, while others sit in a grey area where early research looks promising but large, high-quality studies are still catching up.

This does not make them wrong, but it does mean that informed consent and clear explanations are especially important. To understand whether something is genuinely useful for you, it can help to know what the procedure involves, what it might reveal and how strong the current evidence is. This chapter will help you understand the following:

- What the most commonly offered procedures involve.
- What they may or may not be able to tell you.
- Where the evidence is strong, evolving or uncertain.
- How to ask whether a particular test is relevant for you.

We are going to look at each add-on in detail, as they can significantly impact the overall cost of treatment and are something that will likely be discussed at your initial appointment.

A good clinic will take time to explain how each option works, who it may help and whether it is truly relevant to your situation. They will not rush you, and they will not present anything as essential without strong reasoning.

Where to seek guidance

The HFEA traffic light system can be a helpful guide, offering a simple way to understand the strength of evidence behind each option. The system is designed to take something complex and make it easier for you to navigate. It uses three colours to show how much reliable scientific evidence there is for an add-on:

- Green means there is good-quality evidence that the add-on is likely to be beneficial for certain patients.
- Amber means the evidence is mixed or uncertain, and doctors do not yet know if the add-on genuinely helps.
- Red means there is little or no evidence that the add-on improves outcomes.

The HFEA updates these ratings regularly as new research emerges, making it one of the most accessible ways for patients to understand what may or may not be worthwhile in their individual situation. Alongside the HFEA, international organisations such as the European Society of Human Reproduction and Embryology (ESHRE), the American Society for Reproductive Medicine (ASRM) and the World Health Organization (WHO) also regularly review evidence and publish guidance that shapes fertility care around the world. These organisations provide recommendations on areas such as IVF treatment, embryo transfer, fertility preservation, genetic testing, male fertility and patient safety.

It is important to understand that fertility medicine is constantly evolving. Recommendations can differ slightly between clinics, countries and professional bodies because evidence continues to develop, and fertility treatment is rarely one-size-fits-all. This does not necessarily mean one clinic is right and another is wrong. Often, it reflects the complexity of the science and the reality that experts do not always fully agree.

If you find the different opinions, colour systems or recommendations confusing, that is completely normal. Many people do. A good clinic should be able to talk you through the evidence slowly and clearly, helping you understand why an add-on is being offered, whether it is relevant to your diagnosis and whether it is something you genuinely want to consider.

Access to diagnostic procedures in the UK

In the UK, many of the tests described here are more readily available in private clinics than in NHS settings. NHS fertility services usually focus on investigations and treatments supported by stronger evidence and considered cost-effective at a population level. More detailed diagnostic work is often reserved for specific clinical indications such as recurrent pregnancy loss, suspected fibroids or when someone is already under a specialist fertility team.

> **Radical honesty: The NHS often works on a 'wait and see' model. This can feel frustrating when you are looking for answers early on. Private care may offer more extensive testing, but it also brings financial considerations.**

You are allowed to ask not only 'What can we test?' but also 'What difference will this test make to my care?'

With that in mind, let's look at the procedure you are most likely to encounter: hysteroscopy.

Hysteroscopy

A hysteroscopy involves passing a thin camera through the cervix to look directly inside the uterus. It may be:

- diagnostic, to identify polyps, fibroids, scarring or a septum; or
- operative, where treatment such as polyp removal is carried out at the same time.

Depending on the setting and purpose, a hysteroscopy can be performed under local or general anaesthetic. Most people go home the same day and resume normal activity within a day or two.

Evidence

The evidence for hysteroscopy is strong when there is a clear suspicion of a problem inside the uterus. Identifying these problems matters, because removing polyps, fibroids that distort the uterus, or scar tissue can improve outcomes. However, the treatment usually happens in a separate operative hysteroscopy, not during the initial diagnostic procedure. The first hysteroscopy is often simply to confirm what is there and to plan what needs to happen next.

> **Radical honesty: Hysteroscopy can be transformative when there is a structural concern.**

After looking at the physical environment of the uterus, some clinics turn their attention to timing. Even when the uterus appears healthy, there can still be uncertainty about whether the lining is receptive at the exact moment an embryo is placed. Endometrial receptivity array (ERA) is one of the tests designed to explore this.

Endometrial receptivity array (ERA)

ERA examines gene activity in the uterine lining to estimate when it is most receptive to an embryo. The idea is that not everyone's window of implantation falls at the same time.

It usually involves a mock cycle that mirrors an FET cycle (*see* pp. 180–84). Instead of transferring an embryo, a small biopsy is taken and analysed. If the lining appears pre-receptive or post-receptive, the timing of your real transfer may be adjusted by a day or two.

Who might benefit

ERA is not usually recommended after a single failed transfer. It may be considered when several good-quality embryos have failed to implant despite a normal-looking uterus.

> **Radical honesty: ERA can feel reassuring because it suggests personalised timing. However, the science is evolving, and ERA's impact on live birth rates is still uncertain.**

A helpful question is: 'If this changes my timing, how much difference might it realistically make for someone like me?'

If ERA shows that your timing needs a small adjustment, this can often be addressed quite simply in a future treatment cycle. But if timing alone does not explain previous outcomes, the next question becomes the environment the embryo is meeting. Endometrial microbiome analysis (EMMA) is the test used to explore the microbiome that shapes that environment.

Endometrial microbiome analysis (EMMA)

EMMA examines the bacterial environment within the uterine lining. A sample of fluid or tissue is taken and analysed to identify the bacteria present. If an imbalance is detected, treatment might include antibiotics, probiotics or other approaches to support a healthier microbiome.

> **Radical honesty: Research into the reproductive microbiome is promising but early. We do not yet have strong evidence that testing and treating the microbiome consistently improves live birth rates. EMMA may be helpful in complex cases but is not essential for everyone.**

In some cases, even if the microbiome looks settled, there can still be questions about why implantation has not happened as hoped. For some people, this leads to a different line of enquiry altogether: the role of the immune system. This is where discussions about immunological testing sometimes begin.

Immunological testing

Immunological testing explores whether the immune system might be affecting implantation or pregnancy. It looks at how your body responds to an embryo at the cellular and inflammatory level. Tests may include those listed below:

- Natural killer (NK) cells
- Antiphospholipid antibodies
- Autoantibodies
- Cytokine patterns

This area is both promising and complex. Some clinics use these tests routinely, while others avoid them almost entirely. The variation in approach reflects ongoing debate and the fact that large-scale evidence is still catching up with what many clinicians and patients observe in practice.

A clearer way to understand the immune approach

One of the guiding ideas behind reproductive immunology is that an embryo is genetically unique. Half of its DNA comes from you, and the other half comes from your partner (the same principle is true if you are using donor eggs or sperm). To the immune system, this can look like something unfamiliar. In most pregnancies, the immune system adapts and supports implantation without difficulty. However, the theory is that in some cases, this adjustment does not happen easily. The immune system behaves as if it needs to protect you, triggering inflammation or interrupting the process. Immune therapy aims to calm specific responses during the time an embryo is trying to implant, helping the body welcome something that is biologically different rather than defend against it.

There are a number of situations where immune testing is clearly relevant:

- Recurrent pregnancy loss with suspected antiphospholipid syndrome.
- Known autoimmune conditions such as lupus.
- Unexplained clotting problems.

In these situations, blood tests may show raised immune or clotting markers. Treatment does not aim to switch off the immune system; instead, it aims to calm specific pathways that may be overactive during implantation. The goal is to reduce inflammation, improve blood flow and create an environment where the embryo is more likely to settle and grow.

When there is a clearly identified clotting condition such as antiphospholipid syndrome, this approach is well recognised and can meaningfully improve outcomes. This sits firmly within established reproductive care.

Where things become more controversial is in broader immune profiling when there is no formal autoimmune diagnosis. Tests for NK cells, cytokine balance or other immune markers do not yet have standard reference ranges on which everyone agrees. Different laboratories use different thresholds, and interpretation can vary between clinicians.

This does not mean the science is incorrect; rather, it means the field is still developing and research is ongoing.

> **Radical honesty: We support immune approaches when used thoughtfully. Not as a blanket fix, not as a guarantee and not as something you should feel pushed towards, but as a genuine option worth considering – especially when repeated implantation failure or loss leaves you wondering what else might be contributing.**

Immune treatment can be a powerful part of a personalised plan. It can also be an expensive detour if used without clear purpose.

When immune investigations have been explored, the focus sometimes shifts from the environment in which an embryo tries to implant to the embryo's own genetic health. It is natural to wonder whether the embryos themselves might hold part of the story. This is where PGT can be helpful, offering insight into the chromosomal or genetic make-up of an embryo before transfer.

Preimplantation genetic testing (PGT)

PGT refers to genetic screening carried out on embryos created through IVF *before* they are transferred into the uterus. The aim is simple: to give clearer information about the chromosomes or specific genes within an embryo, so that your clinical team can make more informed and personalised decisions about which embryo has the best chance of leading to a healthy pregnancy.

> **Radical honesty: Most often, the decision comes down to finances, as PGT can add significant cost to a treatment cycle. While it may not increase your overall chance of pregnancy, it can reduce the risk of pregnancy loss.**

Types of PGT

PGT is an umbrella term that covers several types of testing. Each one offers something slightly different and is used for different clinical reasons.

PGT-A

PGT-A looks at the number of chromosomes in an embryo. Chromosomes carry all of our genetic material, and having too many or too few can affect implantation, increase the chance of pregnancy loss or lead to certain chromosomal conditions.

This testing does not 'guarantee' a baby, but it can help prioritise which embryos are most likely to develop normally.

PGT-M

PGT-M is used when a specific inherited condition is already known within the family, such as cystic fibrosis or sickle cell disease.

This test looks for that exact gene change, so the team can identify which embryos are unaffected.

PGT-SR

PGT-SR is used when one partner carries a known structural rearrangement of chromosomes, such as a balanced translocation (*see* p. 49). These rearrangements can sometimes make it harder for embryos to develop normally.

PGT-SR helps identify which embryos have a balanced or normal chromosome pattern.

PGT-P

PGT-P (polygenic testing) is a newer and more complex form of testing. Rather than looking for a single chromosome error or a specific gene, it looks at many genes at once to estimate the likelihood of certain multifactorial conditions.

At the time of writing, PGT-P is not widely used in the UK and is not recommended by many clinics or regulators, including the HFEA. This is because the evidence is still limited and ethical considerations are significant.

What actually happens in PGT

During IVF, embryos are usually cultured in the laboratory for five to six days until they reach the blastocyst stage. At this point, a tiny number of cells are gently removed from the part of the embryo that will eventually become the placenta. The embryo is then frozen and safely stored, and the biopsy sample is sent to a specialist genetics laboratory for analysis.

This is called an embryo biopsy. The sample cells are examined to understand whether the embryo has the correct number of chromosomes, whether it carries a known inherited condition or whether there is a structural genetic issue the family is already aware of.

What PGT can and cannot tell you

PGT does not scan the entire genome. It is not a full genetic map of the embryo. What it can give you is information about the following points:

- Whether the embryo has the expected number of chromosomes.
- Whether it carries a specific inherited condition that is known in the family.
- Whether there is a structural chromosome rearrangement (such as a translocation).
- Depending on the type of test, whether an embryo is more likely to implant and develop normally.

Clinics will often use terms like 'euploid', 'aneuploid' or 'mosaic' in relation to PGT:

- Euploid embryos have the usual number of chromosomes.
- Aneuploid embryos have extra or missing chromosomes.
- Mosaic embryos contain a mixture of normal and abnormal cells.

Mosaic embryos are a developing area of research. Some mosaic embryos can still lead to healthy pregnancies, but the chances can vary, and the risk of pregnancy loss may be higher. Your clinic should explain this slowly, clearly and with nuance if mosaic results appear in your report.

Who PGT is usually offered to

PGT-M and PGT-SR are generally offered when there is a very clear reason: for example, when there is a known genetic condition in the family or when one partner carries a balanced translocation. These tests have strong evidence behind them and can meaningfully reduce the chance of passing on a serious illness.

PGT-A is more complex. It is sometimes considered in the following scenarios:

- There have been recurrent pregnancy losses.
- There have been repeated failed transfers despite good-quality embryos.
- There are many embryos and you are choosing which to transfer first.
- Age or egg quality raises questions about chromosomal health.

In the UK, PGT-A is not recommended as standard for everyone. The evidence does not support universal use.

And then there is PGT-P. As noted earlier, this is still emerging and sits in a controversial space ethically and clinically. At present, many regulators (including the UK's HFEA and most international bodies) advise caution.

What the evidence actually says

For PGT-M and PGT-SR, the evidence is firm and reassuring. These tests absolutely help families to avoid passing on conditions they already know they carry.

For PGT-A, the evidence is mixed. Some groups benefit. Others see no difference in outcome. Professional bodies, including the HFEA and the American Society for Reproductive Medicine (ASRM), advise that PGT-A may help in certain clearly defined situations but should not be treated as a guarantee or a cure-all.

It is also important to remember: PGT cannot 'fix' an embryo. It cannot add missing chromosomes or remove extra ones. It can only tell you what is already there.

For some people, that knowledge prevents the heartbreak of transferring an embryo with no real chance of developing. For others, it simply adds cost, time and emotional pressure without changing the final outcome. Before deciding, it can help to ask yourself these questions:

- *What exactly will this test change for me?*
- *Would the results influence my decisions?*
- *How will I cope if the results are uncertain or unexpected?*
- *Does the cost feel justified at this stage of my journey?*

The emotional side of PGT no one prepares you for

People are often surprised by how intense PGT results feel. Even when you know logically that not every embryo will be chromosomally normal, seeing the words 'abnormal', 'no result' or 'not suitable for transfer' can feel like a deep loss.

We have sat with many patients through this moment. It can be unbelievably painful. These are not just clusters of cells to you. These are possibilities. Futures. Potential babies. And to lose them before the journey even begins can feel deeply unfair.

Please know that you are not alone if you find this part harder than you expected.

Next, we will move into some of the laboratory techniques clinics may offer alongside PGT and explore them with the same radically honest, patient-centred perspective you deserve.

Assisted hatching

Assisted hatching involves creating a tiny opening in the outer shell of the embryo to help it break out before implantation. It may be considered when previous transfers have not been successful or when the shell appears thicker than usual. The evidence for improved outcomes is inconsistent, and both HFEA and ESHRE classify assisted hatching as amber or red depending on the context. It may help some people, but it is not used routinely.

Embryo glue

Embryo glue is a transfer medium containing hyaluronic acid, intended to support adhesion between embryo and uterus. Some clinics use it as standard practice, while others use it only in specific cases such as repeated implantation failure. The evidence suggests a possible benefit, but it is not strong enough to confirm universal improvement. HFEA currently lists it as amber.

As technology has progressed, attention has also turned to how embryos develop within the laboratory itself.

Time-lapse incubators

Systems such as EmbryoScope allow embryos to grow in a stable environment with continuous imaging. This reduces handling and provides detailed insight into development, which can be helpful when selecting embryos.

However, research has not consistently shown that time-lapse incubation increases live birth rates compared with standard methods. It enhances observation rather than guaranteeing improved outcomes.

Closely linked to this is the medium in which embryos grow.

Embryo culture medium variations

Different clinics may use enriched or alternative media designed to nurture early embryo growth. These differences can reflect lab preference, philosophy or evolving research. Current evidence is promising but not decisive, suggesting that outcomes relate more to overall laboratory quality than to one specific media type.

After exploring embryo development, some people move to questions about the environment to which the embryo is transferred.

Uterine NK cell biopsy

A uterine NK cell biopsy involves taking a small sample from the lining of the uterus to measure immune activity at the implantation site. It is very different from blood NK and cytokine testing, which we do believe can offer useful information for some patients when interpreted carefully. The uterine biopsy itself sits in a very uncertain area of fertility medicine.

> **Radical honesty: There is still no agreed 'normal range' and no universal guidelines, and results vary depending on timing and the laboratory. But the evidence is still growing.**

This does *not* make the test harmful; it simply means the evidence is limited at the time of writing. If it is ever suggested to you, a grounding question to ask is: 'How will this result change my treatment in a real, practical way?'

Let's now look at some exciting advancements.

AI tools for eggs, sperm and embryos

AI is becoming more common in embryology laboratories, not as a replacement for skilled scientists but as an extra analytical layer that can spot patterns too subtle for the human eye. These systems review images of eggs, sperm and embryos, looking for clues that may help guide decisions during treatment.

Eggs

AI programmes can analyse features such as the outer layer of the egg, the appearance of the cytoplasm and signs of maturity. These insights may help predict which eggs are more likely to fertilise, although this area is still developing.

Sperm

AI systems can assess sperm shape, movement and behaviour in real time. Because they can process thousands of data points at once, they may give a more detailed picture than manual observation alone, sometimes helping embryologists (the highly trained scientists who care for your embryos in the laboratory and assess how they are developing) choose sperm for ICSI (*see* pp. 184–85).

Embryos

Time-lapse incubators photograph embryos as they grow. AI models then evaluate patterns in cell division and development. Many clinics now use AI scoring alongside the embryologist's own assessment to add another viewpoint, not to replace expertise.

Radical honesty: AI is an exciting tool, but right now it offers information, not certainty. It does not increase pregnancy chances on its own, and research on whether it improves live birth rates is still evolving.

At this time, we like to think of AI as supportive, not decisive, technology that may help you and your team feel more informed.

Calcium ionophore activation

Calcium ionophore activation is sometimes offered after repeated failed fertilisation in ICSI cycles. It helps mimic the natural calcium surge that normally occurs when a sperm successfully activates an egg.

It is not a routine add-on and should not be used broadly. The strongest evidence supports its use only when fertilisation failure has happened more than once, and usually in the context of clear fertilisation problems.

Platelet-rich plasma (PRP)

PRP is appearing more frequently in fertility settings, although it is still considered experimental. It involves taking a sample of your own blood, concentrating the platelets and reintroducing them into the uterus or ovaries. Platelets carry growth factors that may support healing, increase blood flow and encourage tissue repair. The idea is not to add something foreign but to work with your own biology.

There are two main approaches you might come across.

PRP for a thin uterine lining

Some clinics offer PRP when the endometrium does not thicken well despite standard medication. Infusing PRP into the uterus may help the lining grow by supporting regeneration and improving circulation. A number of small studies and patient reports describe positive changes, although results vary and the evidence is still developing. For some, it makes a noticeable difference. For others, the lining remains resistant, even after treatment.

PRP for ovarian support

When injected into the ovaries, PRP is sometimes described as 'ovarian rejuvenation'. The aim is to encourage follicle development or improve the response to stimulation. Early research suggests there may be changes in hormone levels or follicle activity in some cases. However, PRP has not been proven to restore ovarian function or reverse age-related decline, and expectations need to remain gentle and realistic.

Radical honesty: PRP is becoming more widely discussed in fertility treatment, particularly for patients with limited options, but the evidence remains limited and uncertain. At present, there is not enough high-quality research to show that PRP reliably improves pregnancy or live birth rates. Some clinics offer it because the procedure appears relatively low risk, but low risk does not automatically mean proven benefit. It is important that patients understand this distinction clearly before deciding whether it is something they wish to pursue.

High-quality studies are still needed before PRP can be considered established practice.

NAD+ (nicotinamide adenine dinucleotide)

NAD+ therapy is one of the newer complementary treatments that some people explore when preparing for fertility treatment. NAD+ is a molecule found in every cell of the body that plays a critical role in energy production, DNA repair and cellular resilience, all of which essential for the development of healthy eggs, sperm and embryos.

As we age, our natural NAD+ levels decline. This drop is thought to contribute to reduced egg quality and sperm function. Emerging studies and anecdotal reports suggest that supplementing with NAD+, whether through oral supplements or IV infusions, may help improve mitochondrial function, enhance cellular energy, stabilise chromosomes and reduce oxidative stress.

While it is not a guaranteed fix, and certainly no substitute for the foundations of fertility health like sleep, nutrition and emotional wellbeing, NAD+ therapy offers an interesting option for those looking to optimise every aspect of their pre-treatment preparation.

Radical honesty: NAD supplements and infusions are attracting attention in fertility and longevity medicine because they are linked to cellular energy and ageing pathways. The science is interesting, but at the moment there is still very limited high-quality evidence showing that NAD improves egg quality, embryo quality or live birth rates in humans. Some clinics and wellness companies market NAD in ways that can sound more certain than the evidence currently supports. It is important to understand that 'promising' does not always mean 'proven,' especially in fertility care where hope can easily outpace the science.

Closing thoughts

In 1978, when the first IVF baby was born, the world responded with a mix of wonder and fear. Scientists were called 'Frankenstein', headlines warned of unnatural science and people questioned whether IVF should exist at all. Yet today, it is one of the most trusted, regulated and transformative medical treatments available. Millions of children are here because of it. What was once misunderstood is now mainstream.

We share this because every new development in reproductive medicine goes through the same cycle: curiosity, critique, cautious excitement and, eventually, clarity. New ideas always sit in that in-between space where potential and uncertainty overlap. That does not make them right or wrong; it simply makes them *new*.

The same is true for laboratory add-ons, AI tools, evolving embryology techniques and emerging ways of understanding eggs, sperm and embryos. Some are essential for specific situations. Some show promise but need stronger evidence. Others add cost and emotional pressure without clear benefit. You do not need to decide quickly. You do not need to agree to anything you do not fully understand. And you do not need to navigate complex information alone.

Our hope is that patients like you are far more informed.

As you move forward, we invite you to keep returning to one grounding question: 'What is the likely benefit of this, for someone with my age, my diagnosis, my embryos and my history, at this point in my journey?' If your clinic can answer that question clearly, you are in safe hands. If they cannot, you are absolutely entitled to keep asking until the answer makes sense.

Bringing it all together

You will have noticed by now that there is no single, neat pathway through fertility treatment. Treatment continually reshapes itself as new information arrives, hormone levels change, scans reveal something new and a previous treatment cycle teaches us how your body responds.

And treatment sits alongside NHS criteria, private options, finances, work schedules, travel, relationships, emotional capacity and the realities of everyday life. Some options may feel like a natural fit. Others may feel heavy, complex or simply not right. All of this makes sense.

So, let's pause for a moment.

Fertility treatment can move you forwards. It can also stir up doubt, hope, frustration, relief, grief, courage and quiet strength, sometimes all in the same week. You may not feel ready the moment something is offered. You may want more time, you may want to move faster, you may change your mind. You get to take this at the pace that feels manageable for you.

This book is here to return to whenever you need it. So, take what helps today, and leave the rest on the page until another moment. In the following chapter, we are going to take a deep dive into fertility medications: which ones you'll come across, what they are and why your clinic may ask you to take them.

When you're ready, that is where we will go next.

10

Fertility protocols and medications used during treatments

In earlier chapters, we explored the different fertility treatments and procedures you may encounter. This chapter focuses on the protocols and medications that are commonly used during those treatments, including what they are and why they are recommended and prescribed. A protocol is essentially the treatment plan: the structure, timing and sequence of medications and steps designed specifically for you. Medications sit *within* a protocol, but the protocol itself is the roadmap, outlining when to start, when to stop, how doses may change and how your body will be monitored along the way.

By this stage, you very likely already have a list of medications in front of you that can feel overwhelming. There may be words like gonadotrophins, progesterone, letrozole, aspirin, Clexane or trigger injections written on a protocol that was explained quickly, in a busy clinic, at the end of a long appointment. You may have nodded, taken the paperwork and walked away thinking, *I have no idea what half of this actually means!*

This chapter is for that moment.

Our intention is to give you clear, human explanations regarding the usual medications you may come across during your fertility journey, so that when someone says, 'We are going to start you on this protocol' and 'We are going to start you on this medicine', you understand what it does, why it is being suggested and what questions you might want to ask.

You will meet several categories of medication. We will move through them one at a time, calmly and without rush, before finishing with practical advice on how to take your medications.

But first, it helps to understand in more detail what clinicians mean when they talk about protocols.

Stimulation protocols

A stimulation protocol is a treatment plan that guides how and when you take medication to stimulate your ovaries. The goal is to help more than one egg mature, so that several can be collected, fertilised and developed into embryos.

Protocols look different for different people. Your clinic may recommend one based on your age, ovarian reserve, previous treatment and how your hormones behave at baseline. Some clinics will monitor a complete menstrual cycle first to understand this baseline, while others will begin treatment without that additional step. You may hear unfamiliar protocol names along the way. They often sound more complex than they are: most protocols follow the same core stages you will read about in this chapter.

Here is a simple overview of the main IVF stimulation protocols. You do not need to remember them now, unless you want to. They are here to return to if your clinic mentions one of them directly to you.

Agonist-based stimulation cycles

Agonist medications such as buserelin, Lupron or Decapeptyl work by first stimulating and then gradually quietening the pituitary gland. When used continuously, they create a controlled hormonal environment. The deep suppression gives clinicians a high level of control, but it can also cause temporary menopausal symptoms. Hot flushes, night sweats, low mood, headaches and vaginal dryness are all common. While temporary, these sensations can feel unsettling, and many people describe this stage as emotionally demanding.

The long agonist protocol

This is one of the most traditional IVF approaches. Treatment begins in the luteal phase, usually about a week before your period (*see* p. 18). By the time your period arrives, the pituitary gland is switched off and stimulation with FSH or human menopausal gonadotrophin (hMG) begins. This protocol is excellent for preventing premature ovulation. It may be suggested for people with endometriosis (*see* pp. 36–39), fibroids or complex hormonal patterns. However, the suppression phase is longer and can feel heavier both physically and emotionally. For some, particularly those with low ovarian reserve, it may be less suitable.

Follicular phase downregulation

This variation of the long agonist protocol begins at the start of the period rather than in the previous menstrual cycle. The aim is the same: to quieten natural hormones before stimulation begins. It offers timing flexibility for people who need to start quickly or who present later in a cycle. The experience is similar to the long agonist protocol, including the temporary menopausal effects, but the timeline can be more adaptable.

The flare or microdose protocol

The flare protocol uses agonists in a different way. A very small dose is given at the beginning of the menstrual cycle to create a brief release of FSH and LH, known as a flare. This can be especially useful for people with low ovarian reserve, where every follicle counts. After this initial surge, stimulation continues with gonadotrophins. It requires careful monitoring, as the flare can cause overstimulation in the wrong situation, but for those who have responded poorly before, it can make a meaningful difference.

Antagonist-based stimulation cycles

Antagonist medications such as Cetrotide, Orgalutran or Fyremadel act immediately to block the LH surge and prevent premature ovulation. Because suppression is not required beforehand, antagonist cycles are shorter and often easier to tolerate.

Stimulation usually begins on day two or three of the menstrual cycle, and the antagonist is introduced only once follicles are growing. This follows the body's natural rhythm more closely, which is one reason antagonist cycles are now commonly used worldwide.

Many people feel physically and emotionally better on this approach, as there is no downregulation phase and menopausal symptoms are avoided. The risk of OHSS is also lower, especially when a gentler trigger is used. Antagonist cycles are often the first-line approach for new IVF patients, for those with PMOS (*see* pp. 30–31) or high response and for anyone wanting a shorter and more manageable experience.

Mild or mini stimulation

This protocol uses lower doses of injectable medications, sometimes combined with clomifene or letrozole. The focus is not on high egg numbers but on quality. This option can be helpful for older women, those with low ovarian reserve or those who prefer fewer injections. While egg numbers are often lower, some people find it physically and emotionally gentler.

Letrozole-based stimulation

This approach reduces oestrogen levels and can reduce the risk of OHSS. Often used in people with PMOS, in breast cancer patients or as part of mild stimulation, it can also be used in natural cycle IVF (*see* p. 216).

Progestin-primed ovarian stimulation (PPOS)

PPOS uses oral progesterone tablets rather than an antagonist to prevent the LH surge. This can be useful for egg accumulation or repeated treatment cycles. The lining is affected by progesterone, so transfer is delayed and embryos are frozen for later.

DuoStim (double stimulation in one cycle)

This protocol stimulates the ovaries twice in one menstrual cycle: first in the follicular phase and again in the luteal phase (*see* p. 18). This can be valuable for people with very low ovarian reserve or for urgent fertility preservation (*see* pp. 185–86). Eggs and embryos are usually frozen after each collection.

Luteal-phase stimulation alone

Stimulation can begin after ovulation and still produce eggs of similar quality. This offers flexibility when timing is limited.

Back-to-back cycles

Back-to-back cycles entail beginning a stimulation cycle immediately after egg collection. This approach is useful when the goal is to accumulate eggs quickly or where ovarian reserve is low.

Natural cycle IVF

Natural cycle IVF relies on the body's own follicles and does not use stimulation. It is often used when medication does not increase egg yield or when a minimal intervention approach feels more aligned.

Start any time protocols

Modern IVF is increasingly flexible. Some clinics can start treatment cycles outside of the usual day one or day two framework, which helps in urgent situations or where someone's schedule needs accommodation.

Every stimulation protocol is a tool. No one protocol is always best, and none of them define your likelihood of becoming a parent. The right protocol is the one that matches your biology, your history and your emotional needs. Understanding why a particular approach is suggested turns IVF from something that is done to you into something you are part of. When the plan makes sense, treatment often feels less overwhelming and more grounded.

How are you doing so far? There is lots of information to take in, we know. With that in mind, let's move onto the medication that supports these protocols.

We begin where most people begin: with stimulation of the ovaries.

Medicines that stimulate the ovaries

A brief science moment. In a natural menstrual cycle, the brain releases two key hormones called FSH and LH. They travel to the ovaries and encourage one follicle to grow and release a mature egg. IVF changes this rhythm on purpose.

Instead of hoping for a single egg each month, treatment aims to support the ovaries to produce several eggs so that embryos can be created and chosen carefully. The medicines used in this phase are not foreign to your body. They amplify signals the ovaries already know how to follow.

These medicines are usually injectable and contain either FSH alone or a combination of FSH and LH. Each does a similar job, with small differences depending on what your clinic feels you need.

FSH injections

FSH medicines are often the starting point of stimulation. They usually come as small injections given just under the skin of the tummy or thigh. FSH encourages follicles to grow and develop. Many people give these once a day, although some protocols use twice-daily doses.

FSH and LH combination injections

Some stimulation medicines contain both FSH and LH, and are sometimes called hMG or menotrophins. Clinics may choose these when they feel both hormones together will support healthy follicle development.

What you may notice

Some people feel bloated, heavy or tender around the pelvis as follicles grow. Others feel very little change. Emotionally, you might notice that keeping track of doses, scans and timings takes up energy. This is normal. Many people end up injecting themselves in the bathroom at work or in their car between other commitments.

Subcutaneous injections

Subcutaneous means the medication is delivered just under the skin rather than into muscle. The needles are very fine, and, with practice, injections often feel more manageable than people expect. They tend to become a familiar rhythm over time rather than something to fear.

Most commonly, IVF medications are injected into the lower tummy, about two finger-widths away from the belly button. You can also use the upper thigh (*see* p. 228).

> **Radical honesty: The first injection does not always feel calm. You may sit there for a while, gathering yourself. You may need several tries. Many people do. It is an odd thing to inject yourself for the first time, and there is no one right way to arrive at that moment.**

Trigger injection

Towards the end of the stimulation phase, your clinic will ask you to take a trigger injection. It is given in much the same way as the other subcutaneous injections you have been using. This final dose prepares the eggs for collection by mimicking the natural surge of LH that would usually lead to ovulation. Timing is precise. You may be asked to take it at a specific hour so that egg collection can take place at the right moment, usually around 35–37 hours later.

As the follicles mature after the trigger injection, you may notice increased bloating or discomfort. Most of the time, this is expected. However, if you feel severe pain, have difficulty breathing or notice rapid swelling, contact your clinic, as these may be early signs of OHSS (*see* p. 157).

As stimulation progresses, follicles continue to grow under the guidance of these medicines. Clinics monitor this through scans and blood tests, adjusting doses when needed. Once the follicles are developing well, the next step is making sure you do not ovulate too soon.

This is where the second group of medicines plays its part.

Medicines that prevent premature ovulation

While stimulation medicines encourage follicles to grow, another group of medicines is used to prevent ovulation from happening too soon. In a natural menstrual cycle, the body releases an egg when LH rises sharply. During IVF, your clinic will want to guide the timing so that egg collection can take place safely. They do this through medicines that temporarily hold ovulation back, keeping the eggs in the follicles until the right moment.

There are two main types: gonadotrophin-releasing hormone (GnRH) antagonists and GnRH agonists. Their names sound technical, but their purpose is straightforward. They create a pause in the normal hormonal rhythm so the follicles can continue growing without releasing the egg before the clinic is ready.

GnRH antagonists

GnRH antagonists are often started once follicles reach a certain size during stimulation. They act quickly and are usually given as daily injections alongside your FSH or FSH plus LH medicine. Some people notice very little difference while using them. Others describe small shifts in mood or energy. Both experiences are common.

GnRH agonists

GnRH agonists work differently. They first create a brief rise in hormone signals, then suppress them. When they are used as part of a downregulation phase, they lower the natural hormonal rhythm for a short time. Some people describe warm flushes, headaches or irritability during this period. These sensations usually settle as the next stage begins, although you may not notice anything at all.

Downregulation

Some fertility treatment protocols include a short phase called downregulation. This means temporarily quietening or switching off your body's own reproductive hormone signals before stimulation begins.

Downregulation helps your medical team take control of your menstrual cycle, preventing your ovaries from releasing an egg too early and allowing medications to work in a more predictable, coordinated way. You may hear it described as 'putting the ovaries to sleep' or creating a temporary menopause-like state; but it is important to know that this effect is fully reversible.

This phase usually lasts a few days to a few weeks, depending on the protocol being used. Once stimulation medications are started, your ovaries are gently 'woken up' again.

COMMON DRUG NAMES YOU MAY COME ACROSS

- GnRH antagonists: Cetrotide, cetrorelix, ganirelix
- GnRH agonists: buserelin, triptorelin, leuprorelin
- Sometimes used for downregulation or trigger: Decapeptyl
- FSH medications: Gonal-F, Puregon, Bemfola, Ovaleap, Fostimon
- Combined FSH and LH medications: Menopur, Pergoveris, Meriofert, Merional
- Trigger medications: Ovitrelle, Pregnyl, Gonasi, Decapeptyl

As you move through this phase, you are preparing for egg collection. The medicines you have already taken have encouraged follicles to grow. The medicines you take here ensure that growth continues without early release. When the follicles look ready, the next step is the trigger injection we discussed in the previous section (*see* pp. 218–19). After that, the focus moves towards egg collection and, if needed, supporting ovulation or implantation in treatment cycles that do not involve IVF.

In the section ahead, we will look at medicines that are sometimes used outside IVF to encourage ovulation, as well as what they do and how they are chosen.

Medicines used to induce ovulation outside IVF cycles

Not everyone begins treatment with IVF. Sometimes, the first step is helping the body ovulate more predictably. If ovulation is irregular, absent or difficult to track, your clinic may offer medication that encourages the ovary to release an egg. These medicines are often used in timed intercourse cycles or IUI (*see* pp. 177–78), and for some people they lead to pregnancy without needing any further medical support. For others, they provide useful information about how the ovaries respond and what support might be helpful next.

Clomifene citrate

Clomifene works by briefly blocking oestrogen signals in the brain. When the brain senses less oestrogen, it releases more FSH and LH, which can prompt ovulation. Some people ovulate with clomifene when they have not been ovulating regularly on their own.

Side effects can include warm flushes, headaches or irritability, although many people describe nothing noticeable at all. For some, the uterine lining can become thinner when using clomifene, which is one reason clinics may suggest only a set number of treatment cycles. Ultrasound scans are often used to track follicle growth and response.

Letrozole

Letrozole briefly lowers oestrogen production so that FSH rises naturally. It is often used for people with PMOS (*see* pp. 30–31) and may be gentler on the uterine lining than clomifene. It can also be offered if clomifene has not triggered ovulation. Some people feel a little fatigued or light-headed while using it, while others notice very little. As with clomifene, scans are used to monitor response so that ovulation can be timed accurately.

Metformin

Metformin is most commonly used in people with PMOS (*see* pp. 30–31) where insulin resistance may play a role in ovulation. It can support hormone balance, and, in some cases, it helps menstrual cycles to become more regular. Unlike clomifene or letrozole, it is not an ovulation medicine on its own, but it can create a more favourable environment for ovulation to occur. Some people experience stomach upset at the beginning, which often settles as the dose is increased gradually.

Ovulation medicines can feel like a hopeful first step for some people and like another step in a long process for others. If one option does not work for you, it provides more information about what may be needed next. Some people conceive using these medicines, while others move towards IVF feeling clearer and more informed. There is no one path that is more successful or more valid.

If ovulation medicines are not enough on their own, or if treatment moves towards IVF or FET, the focus shifts to supporting implantation and early pregnancy. The medicines in the next section help prepare the lining of the uterus so that an embryo can settle and begin to grow.

Medicines that support implantation and early pregnancy

Once eggs have been collected and fertilised, or when you are preparing for an FET, the focus of medication changes. The aim is no longer to stimulate the ovaries but to prepare and support the lining of the uterus so that an embryo can settle.

Two main hormones play a role here: oestrogen builds and thickens the endometrium, while progesterone stabilises it and supports implantation.

Oestrogen

Oestrogen is often used to prepare the uterine lining before progesterone is introduced. You may be given tablets, patches, gel or spray. Each clinic uses slightly different methods and schedules, though they all work in a similar way: they support the uterine lining to grow so that it becomes receptive to an embryo.

Progesterone

Progesterone supports implantation and early pregnancy. It is started after egg collection or in the days leading up to embryo transfer, depending on whether you are having a fresh or frozen cycle (*see* pp. 181–84). It is usually continued until around the time the placenta begins producing its own hormones. Your clinic will guide you on when to start and how long to continue.

Progesterone can be given in several forms. None is more virtuous or brave than another. The right choice is simply the one you can live with day to day.

Vaginal or rectal progesterone

Many clinics use vaginal progesterone as the first option. Capsules, gels or pessaries placed in the vagina or rectum are absorbed locally through the uterine blood supply. Because the progesterone is absorbed close to where it is needed, blood test levels may look lower than with injections even though the effect on the uterine lining is strong. Vaginal progesterone can feel messy at times, as the base dissolves and returns as discharge. Some people find this manageable; others prefer rectal use, which can feel cleaner or less emotionally charged. Both routes work well.

Oral progesterone

Sometimes used alongside vaginal or rectal forms, oral progesterone supports progesterone levels in the bloodstream. Some people notice tiredness, light dizziness or a sense of sedation after taking it. Others feel very little change.

Subcutaneous progesterone injections

Subcutaneous progesterone is injected just under the skin, usually into the abdomen or thigh, using a smaller needle than intramuscular progesterone. It is designed to provide progesterone support in a way that many people find easier and less painful to manage at home. The medication is absorbed into the bloodstream to help maintain progesterone levels during the luteal phase and early pregnancy support. Some people experience mild stinging, redness or bruising at the injection site, while others find it more comfortable than progesterone in oil injections.

Intramuscular progesterone injections

Intramuscular progesterone, often called progesterone in oil, is given as a deeper injection into muscle rather than under the skin. It is usually injected into the buttock (*see* pp. 228–29 for a how-to guide). The medication is absorbed steadily into the bloodstream, supporting stable progesterone levels. This method can be very effective, although it may feel physically heavier to manage over time.

How you may feel on progesterone

Progesterone influences neurotransmitters linked to emotional regulation. Because treatment doses are often higher than the body would usually produce on its own, some people notice changes in mood. You may feel unusually sensitive, tearful or reactive. Some describe irritability or anxiety. Others feel flat or low in energy, or find that ordinary stress feels heavier than usual. Fatigue is common too, as progesterone has a naturally sedating effect. Not everyone experiences these changes, but if you do, it helps to know that it is a hormonal effect rather than a reflection of how well you are coping.

Progesterone interacts with gamma-aminobutyric acid (GABA) receptors in the brain, which usually promote calm. When GABA levels rise quickly or stay high for long periods, they can temporarily affect emotional steadiness. These shifts tend to settle over time or once treatment transitions. You are responding to chemistry, not failing to cope.

Gentle movement such as walking or stretching can help. Some find slow breathing or short mindfulness practices grounding. Talking openly with someone close, or noting your feelings in writing, can make emotions feel less compressed inside you. You are not required to feel positive. You only need enough space to get through each day.

Radical honesty: Progesterone plays a vital role in supporting implantation and early pregnancy, yet living with it can be demanding. The routines are repetitive and sometimes physically uncomfortable. Mood shifts can arrive without warning. Knowing why it is needed does not always make the experience easier, but it can bring clarity to what is happening in your body.

Adjunct and immune-related medications

Alongside the core medicines that stimulate the ovaries and support implantation, you may come across medications that sit around the edges of a treatment cycle. Some of these are used widely, while others are more selective, used only when the medical team thinks there may be benefit based on your history or blood tests. You are not expected to know which you need. Treatment is not about gathering every option. It is about using what is appropriate for your body, at the right time, with a clear reason.

We will move slowly through the most common adjunct medicines first, then into the immune-modulating treatments that are used more selectively.

You can take your time here; we suggest you do so.

Common adjunct ‘add-on’ medications

Aspirin

Low-dose aspirin (often 75mg) is sometimes used to support blood flow to the uterus and reduce inflammation, particularly in people with recurrent pregnancy loss or suspected immune-related issues. Some people take it throughout stimulation or early pregnancy; others do not need it at all. Your clinic will guide you.

Clexane (enoxaparin)

Clexane is an anticoagulant that reduces the risk of blood clot formation. It may be recommended when clotting factors are raised, when thrombophilia is present or when pregnancy loss or implantation difficulty is thought to have a vascular component. It is given as a small subcutaneous injection, often daily. Bruising is common.

> **Radical honesty: Clexane increases bleeding risk. For some people, the benefit outweighs this; for others, it is not needed. Your clinic should explain how this applies to you.**

Steroids (corticosteroids)

Steroids such as prednisolone may be used to calm inflammatory or immune responses that could interfere with implantation. They are usually taken for a limited time: often up to 12 weeks if pregnancy occurs. Some people notice agitation, restlessness or difficulty sleeping on steroids. These medications require a clear start and stop plan.

Sildenafil

More widely known for other uses, sildenafil (Viagra) is sometimes used to improve uterine blood flow, especially when the lining grows slowly. It may be prescribed orally or as a vaginal pessary. Headaches, flushing or light dizziness can occur.

Cabergoline

Cabergoline is sometimes used around the time of the trigger injection (*see* pp. 218–19) to reduce the risk of OHSS. It lowers prolactin levels and helps prevent fluid shifting into the abdomen. It is usually taken as tablets for a short run of days.

Antibiotics

Antibiotics are not routine, but they may be used if there is concern about infection, in people with past PID or when procedures such as egg collection (*see* pp. 159–60) or hysteroscopy (*see* pp. 199–200) are planned.

Thyroid medication

Thyroid hormones influence ovulation, implantation and early pregnancy. If thyroid levels are outside the desired range, levothyroxine is often prescribed. Dose changes are monitored with blood tests. Many people feel well once dosing stabilises.

You are likely to be offered only the medicines relevant to your situation. Seeing the names here may help you recognise them later, but you do not need to remember them now.

Immune-related medications

Some treatments aim to adjust immune activity when there is suspicion that the immune system may be interacting with implantation or early pregnancy (*see* pp. 52–53). The evidence here is mixed, and views vary between clinics. This does not mean these treatments are ineffective, only that research is ongoing and recommendations are personalised.

These medicines are usually considered when there is a clear trigger such as recurrent pregnancy loss, raised immunity markers, autoimmune conditions or repeated implantation difficulty.

Humira

Humira is a tumour necrosis factor-alpha (TNF-α) inhibitor used widely in autoimmune conditions such as rheumatoid arthritis. In fertility settings, it may be offered when inflammatory markers or NK cell results are raised. It is given as a subcutaneous injection, often before treatment begins, and consent may be required.

Intralipid infusion (ILP)

Intralipids were originally used for nutritional support in people unable to feed orally. In fertility, they are sometimes used to modulate immune response and reduce inflammation, particularly after recurrent pregnancy loss. They are given intravenously in a clinic setting as an infusion.

Intravenous immunoglobulin (IVIG)

IVIG infuses concentrated antibodies to alter immune activity. It may be suggested for recurrent pregnancy loss or suspected immune-mediated implantation problems. Infusions take several hours.

Radical honesty: IVIG is costly, and flu-like symptoms afterwards are common, especially if the treatment is given quickly. Hydrating during the infusion may help.

Lymphocyte immunisation therapy (LIT)

LIT involves injecting white blood cells from the male partner into the female partner's forearm, with the aim of improving immune tolerance of the embryo. It is usually given weeks before treatment and may be repeated.

Radical honesty: LIT is debated within reproductive medicine. Some experience mild skin irritation or swelling afterwards. The evidence base is evolving.

Hydroxychloroquine (HCQ)

HCQ is used for autoimmune conditions such as lupus. In fertility, it may be considered when autoimmune markers are present. It reduces inflammation and helps regulate immune response.

Radical honesty: Short-term HCQ use is generally well tolerated. Longer-term use can affect eyesight, so monitoring is important if used beyond a brief course.

Corticosteroids

Corticosteroids are sometimes used as immune suppressants rather than standard adjunct medication.

If you reach the point where immune-modulating therapy is being discussed, you are not expected to choose blindly or understand every mechanism. This is a point for clear explanation, questions and shared decision-making. You are allowed to ask why a medicine is recommended and what evidence supports it. You are also allowed to pause, think or seek a second opinion if something feels uncertain.

Radical honesty: This is one of the areas in fertility medicine where science, clinical experience and patient hope often overlap. Some patients feel strongly that adjunct medications made a difference to their outcome. Others go through successful treatment without any additional medication at all. The challenge is that fertility research is

complex, and not every potentially helpful treatment has definitive evidence yet. Good clinics should be open about where evidence is strong, where it is still evolving and why they believe a treatment may or may not, be appropriate for you specifically.

Practical guidance for taking your medications

You have now explored the medicines used in treatment, how they work and why they may be suggested. The next part is more practical. It is the moment where medication comes out of the box and into your real life. For many people, this is where treatment becomes tangible. You move from information to action, often in your own home rather than inside the calm of a clinic room.

There is no right way to approach this stage. You do not need to feel brave or organised. You only need to learn what works for you, one dose at a time.

Giving subcutaneous injections

Subcutaneous injections are used for most stimulation medicines, and for Clexane if it is part of your plan. They are given just under the skin, usually in the lower tummy or the upper thigh. The needles are small and fine. Many people feel more nervous before the first injection than during it.

How to give the injection

1. Wash your hands and gather what you need, so nothing feels rushed.
2. Choose an area with soft tissue, often a few finger-widths away from the belly button or on the thigh.
3. Pinch the skin gently between your fingers.
4. Rest the needle against the skin, take a slow breath out and insert the needle at a comfortable angle.
5. Press the plunger slowly, noticing your pace rather than pushing quickly.
6. Pause for a moment before removing the needle.
7. Press lightly with tissue or cotton wool if needed, without rubbing.
8. Place the used needle safely in your sharps bin.

Small things that help

- Let the medication warm slightly towards room temperature. Cold liquid can sting.
- If you hesitate, pause. Touch the needle to your skin first, then breathe out as you begin.
- If your hands shake, sit down. You are allowed to steady yourself.
- You do not have to look if looking is harder. Many inject by feel.

Over time, this may become routine. Not effortless, but familiar.

Giving intramuscular injections

Intramuscular injections, such as progesterone in oil (*see* p. 223), go deeper into the muscle of the buttock. They can feel more physically and emotionally demanding, especially if used over several weeks, but the technique is entirely learnable.

Finding the right place

A gentle visualisation helps. Imagine each buttock divided into four equal squares. The **upper outer square** is the safest injection site. It stays well away from the sciatic nerve which sits deeper and lower. A nurse can show you once if you prefer. Some people mark the area lightly with a washable pen to come back to later.

How to give the injection

1. Sit or stand so the muscle feels relaxed, such as with one foot on a low stool.
2. Hold the skin to steady your hand.
3. Insert the needle slowly and steadily, without force.
4. Inject gradually. Progesterone in oil is thick and responds well to patience.
5. Remove the needle gently, and press the area if you need a moment to steady yourself.
6. Alternate sides with each injection to give the muscle time to recover.
7. A warm compress afterwards can soften the oil and ease tenderness.

Comfort ideas

- Warmth often soothes better than cold afterwards. Some people still prefer a cold pack before to numb the skin. Choose what feels right for you.
- A short walk can ease stiffness. A light massage a few minutes later can help the oil disperse.
- If redness or swelling feels unusual or persists, contact your clinic.

You are not expected to enjoy this. You are only expected to manage what you can, in the way you can.

Managing timings and routine

Medication schedules can look rigid when written on paper, yet real life is fluid. You may find yourself giving an injection in a bathroom at work, in your car or at the kitchen counter before bed. This is not a sign you are doing it badly. This is treatment happening alongside life.

Some people set alarms. Others place their medication beside their toothbrush or kettle. Some keep everything in one basket, so it travels easily from one room to another. If you are travelling, a small cool bag can be helpful. If time zones change, ask your clinic how to adjust gently rather than perfectly.

Organisation is not about aesthetics. It is about reducing stress when things are already being asked of you.

Storing and disposing of medication

Medicines arrive with their own instructions, but some general points apply:

- Many are kept at room temperature unless the label says otherwise.
- Some need refrigeration before mixing.
- Used needles and syringes belong in a sharps bin, not household waste.
- Your clinic or pharmacy can provide replacements if you run low. Feeling stocked and prepared often brings a sense of steadiness.

When things feel emotionally heavy

There may be days when injections feel matter of fact and others when the smallest step feels large. Sometimes, it is not the needle that is painful but the meaning it carries: longing, uncertainty, hope, repetition, waiting. If tears come, they come. You can sit with them. You can still continue after a pause.

You only need to manage one dose at a time. One day at a time. Not the whole treatment at once.

Closing reflection

You have now moved through a landscape of medicines, names, hormones and practical routines. It is a lot to hold on the page, and even more to hold in a body going through treatment. If you feel informed but tired, curious yet full, that is a very natural response.

There will be days when medication feels manageable, and doses and timings fall into place. There may also be days when you hesitate with the needle in your hand or second-guess whether you did something correctly. Many people do both. Learning and uncertainty sit side by side in this process far more often than clarity and confidence do.

If at any point you notice yourself feeling behind, remind yourself that treatment is lived one dose, one appointment, one morning and one evening at a time. You are already doing enough by showing up and asking questions, by pausing to understand and by caring about getting this right for yourself.

As you move on to the next chapter of this book, carry only what feels useful. Leave the rest for now. You can return to it later, in the moment you need it, perhaps with the lid of a sharps bin open beside you or a new prescription sheet on the table.

Take a deep breath: you're doing fantastically.

11

Pregnancy after treatment: early monitoring and the first trimester

Here you are, pregnant! Those words may land with excitement, caution, surprise or something slower. However it feels, we are with you.

The moment you see a positive test

There is often a pause in the moment a pregnancy test turns positive. It does not matter at this stage whether it has happened naturally, through timed intercourse, ovulation medication, IUI or IVF, or after years of trying. Those two lines, or the word 'pregnant', carry a meaning that is specific to you and to everything you have already lived through.

Over the years, when we called patients with a positive blood test for the very first time, we would often say the same thing, 'Go home, do a home pregnancy test and enjoy this feeling.' After months, sometimes years of staring at blank tests, searching for lines that never appeared and bracing for disappointment, this moment deserves to be celebrated. Seeing those two lines after everything it took to get there can feel surreal, emotional and completely overwhelming. Whatever happens next, this is still one of the most special moments in the fertility journey, and you are allowed to feel joy in it.

For some people, the positive test and early pregnancy feel like a rush of joy. For many, it is a mixture of relief, disbelief, hesitation and hope. You may cry within seconds, you may sit very still and keep looking at the test or you may feel nothing at all at first, and only realise later that you felt numb. None of this is a prediction of what will happen next. It is a reflection of your history and everything it has taken to get here.

What we can say with certainty is this. A positive test means that implantation has taken place. An embryo has signalled to your body that it is there, and your hormones have responded. In the background, biological changes begin almost immediately. The embryo starts to organise itself, the very early placenta begins to form and hormone levels rise to protect and support the lining of the uterus.

We have found that physical symptoms vary a great deal. You may notice breast tenderness, tiredness or mild nausea. You may feel completely normal for some time. In our clinical experience, people who conceive after IVF or medicated cycles often report fewer symptoms than those who conceive without treatment. This is because the medications used during treatment can overshadow or mimic the sensations many people expect from early pregnancy. This is one of the most common triggers for early worry, but an absence of symptoms tells us very little about what is happening inside the uterus.

In this chapter, we will stay close to what is actually happening in early pregnancy after treatment. We will look at how pregnancies are monitored, what is usually expected, what can sometimes go wrong and how to navigate the first trimester as calmly as possible, both medically and emotionally.

You are pregnant. For now, it is enough to acknowledge what has begun. Maybe that truth can stand on its own for a moment before anything else is required of you.

When you feel ready to look ahead, it can help to know what the next steps usually involve. Early pregnancy monitoring after treatment has its own rhythm, and we will walk through it together, one stage at a time.

How pregnancy is monitored after treatment

In the first weeks after fertility treatment, you will usually stay under the care of your clinic. This is one of the main differences when conception happens through fertility treatment. In pregnancies conceived without treatment, most people contact their GP early on and wait for their first NHS scan (around 12 weeks of pregnancy). After fertility treatment, the clinic often continues to check in for a short time before care transfers across to the NHS or a private obstetrician. This is routine rather than a sign that anyone expects problems.

What happens in this phase can vary. Some clinics ask you to use a home pregnancy test at home, others arrange blood tests and some continue to check your blood results over a few weeks to make sure that pregnancy hormones are rising. Others move directly to an early ultrasound once pregnancy is confirmed. We hope that your clinic signposts you towards what the next few weeks will look like for you. A plan is often reassuring at this stage, and also gives you something that can anchor you at a time that can feel both hopeful and uncertain.

Many people describe these early weeks as slow. You may notice yourself watching for symptoms or checking whether they come and go, and consulting 'Dr Google' more than you have done before. You might feel okay one day and unsure the next. None of this means anything about the pregnancy itself. Again, this reflects the effort it took to arrive here rather than the pregnancy itself.

You are not expected to do anything except attend the appointments offered and let this part of the process unfold. The next key milestone for most people is the first ultrasound. Understanding what that scan is designed to show can make the waiting feel more manageable.

Your first ultrasound scan

This first ultrasound scan is there to confirm that the pregnancy is developing in the uterus, growing at the expected pace and showing the early signs of progression. At around six weeks, it is common to see the gestational sac or a small bright circle known as the yolk sac. Sometimes, that is all that is visible. The embryo is present but too small to be seen with clarity.

A heartbeat often becomes visible slightly later. For some, this happens near the end of the sixth week. For others, it is closer to seven weeks or beyond. A few days can make a noticeable difference. Timing matters more than most people realise.

Radical honesty: It is possible that you will not see a heartbeat at the first scan. This does not always mean something is wrong. It is early. A repeat scan is usually arranged, and the embryo may grow enough in that time for more to be seen.

If your scan takes place a little later, you may see the flicker of cardiac activity. It is small and quick, and sometimes astonishing to witness.

We have seen people respond in many ways. Some cry, some smile quietly, some are holding their breath so tightly the news almost does not resonate and some feel relief that lasts only until the next wait begins. All of these reactions make sense.

If more than one embryo implants

Sometimes, an early scan shows more than one gestational sac. This means you may be carrying twins or a higher-order multiple pregnancy. Some people feel excitement. Others feel shock, or a mixture of both emotions. You may need time to process what this means for your pregnancy, your body and the months ahead.

Multiple pregnancies are monitored more closely because the physical demands are greater and the chance of complications is slightly higher. Your clinical team will guide you through this and offer additional appointments as needed. You do not have to learn everything at once. In the early weeks, the focus is on confirming development and giving you time to adjust to the idea of more than one baby.

After the scan, the next question is often how far along you are. Knowing your exact treatment dates can make the standard way in which pregnancy is measured feel confusing at first. Understanding how weeks are counted can help the rest of the journey make more sense.

How pregnancy weeks are counted after treatment

One of the first practical questions after a positive test is how far along you are. When conception happens naturally, pregnancy is dated from the first day of the last menstrual period, even though fertilisation usually takes place around two weeks later. After fertility treatment, when you know the exact day of ovulation, insemination, egg collection or embryo transfer, this system can feel counterintuitive.

Even in IVF and IUI pregnancies, the same dating method is used. Pregnancy is still measured from an estimated menstrual cycle start rather than from the day the embryo was created or transferred.

In practice, this means that by the time you see a positive pregnancy test, you are usually counted as being around four weeks pregnant. The embryo may have only been in your body for a short time, but medically you are already about four weeks into the pregnancy calendar.

If you had IUI, the insemination date is treated like ovulation. To match natural conception dating, we count back roughly two weeks and begin from there.

If you had IVF, timing is calculated using the age of the embryo at transfer. For example:

- A fresh cycle counts egg collection as ovulation day.
- A frozen day five blastocyst transfer is counted as if ovulation had occurred five days earlier.

From this point, pregnancy progresses along the usual 40-week timeline that maternity services use.

> **Radical honesty: When your care transfers back into the NHS system, you may find that your dates do not align neatly. Many NHS services use the traditional 'last period' method of calculation. Even when you know the exact day of transfer or insemination, they may still work from the standard chart. This can feel frustrating, especially when you have been living with your dates for weeks.**

You do not need to memorise formulas or calculate anything yourself. Your clinic will guide you, and later your midwife will continue the timeline. What matters most is this: your pregnancy has begun, you are moving forwards week by week and the numbers will fall into place as you go.

With dating understood, we can look at what early development tends to look like from here.

The first trimester week by week

The following timeline is a way to understand what is happening inside your body as the pregnancy develops.

Weeks 4 to 5: the very beginning

Testing usually happens around this time. Medically, you are only days beyond implantation, yet the pregnancy is counted as four to five weeks. Hormone levels are increasing and the embryo is beginning to settle in. You may notice breast tenderness, tiredness or mild nausea, or you may feel nothing at all.

Week 6: a quiet stage of development

Inside your uterus, the foundations of the heart, brain and spinal column are forming within the embryo. The early placenta is organising itself. If your clinic offers a scan at this point, you may see the gestational sac or the yolk sac. It may be too early to see anything more, but a few days can change what is visible.

Week 7: the possibility of the first heartbeat

Many people see the first flicker of cardiac activity during this week or soon after. It is tiny and fast. Seeing it can bring relief, surprise or emotion that is hard to put into words. You may leave the scan room feeling lighter, or you may leave with relief mixed with caution; both make sense.

Week 8: growth, but not always symptoms

The embryo is now about the size of a raspberry. Its brain development is rapid. You might notice tiredness, nausea or changes in appetite. You might still feel very normal. IVF medication can mask or mimic early pregnancy symptoms, and absence of symptoms is common.

Week 9: a subtle transition

Around this time, the embryo becomes clinically known as a fetus. It is a quiet but meaningful shift in development. Your hormone levels are often peaking, which can amplify tiredness and emotional sensitivity. Some people begin to imagine ahead more easily, while others remain very measured. Neither response says anything about attachment or outcome.

Week 10: structure is in place

By week 10, the foundations of organs and limbs are formed. Growth and refinement continue from here. Some people describe feeling slightly more anchored at this point, even if they are not yet secure. Confidence in pregnancy usually increases gradually, not all at once.

Weeks 11–12: approaching the first milestone

Your uterus begins to rise from the pelvis. The fetus can move and swallow, though you will not usually feel movement yet. The first NHS scan often happens around this time. It is a significant appointment for many.

As you move through these early weeks, another part of monitoring may be discussed alongside scans, and that is blood work. Knowing what these results mean can help protect you from unnecessary worry and guide you in deciding how much information feels helpful to you.

Blood tests and hormone monitoring

Not everyone will have blood tests in early pregnancy, but we want to prepare you in case your clinic offers them. Some clinics check hormones once or twice after a positive test. Others move straight to an ultrasound. Both approaches are what we could consider standard practice.

The pregnancy hormone most commonly monitored is hCG. You may also hear the term beta hCG. This is simply the laboratory name for the specific form of the hormone measured in blood tests. hCG is released by the developing placenta after implantation. A positive home pregnancy test means hCG is present. A blood test, if offered, measures the exact amount.

Sometimes, this test is repeated after 48–72 hours. What matters is not the number itself but the pattern. Very roughly, we hope to see the level increase over time, often doubling within that window. A single result tells us very little. A rising trend is usually the reassuring part.

Some clinics also monitor progesterone. As we discussed earlier (*see* p. 18), progesterone supports the lining of the uterus and helps maintain early pregnancy. Testing can guide whether adjustments are needed, but in most cases, medication continues as planned regardless of the exact number. Levels can fluctuate naturally, and a variation of around 40mmol per test is usually not concerning. We tend to look for stability rather than a continuous increase, adjusting treatment only when levels fall outside the expected range.

Radical honesty: It is natural to want certainty, and numbers can feel like certainty. It can be tempting to compare results with other people or to search for charts online. Unfortunately, there is no magic number that guarantees a healthy pregnancy. We have seen low initial levels lead to good outcomes, as well as high starting values that did not continue. Hormone monitoring can reassure, but it can also increase anxiety. It is reasonable to ask your clinic what they hope to learn from each test and how any result will change your care.

For most people, blood tests are used for a short time only. Once an early scan shows that the pregnancy is developing in the right place, with appropriate growth and a heartbeat, ongoing care gradually moves towards routine antenatal pathways.

As monitoring continues, you may notice that progress is measured in small steps. A rising hormone level. A scan that shows what we would hope to see for that point in time. These moments can bring reassurance, yet early pregnancy still involves waiting. It is normal to feel better some days and unsure on others.

It can help to understand what happens when things are progressing as expected. It can also help to know what may go wrong. You are welcome to pause here if this does not feel like the right moment. You can return whenever you want to. If you choose to read on, we will approach this with clarity and compassion.

When things feel uncertain and what may go wrong

Most pregnancies continue as expected. Hormones rise, the scan shows what we hope to see and, week by week, the embryo grows. Even so, the early weeks can feel fragile. When you have worked hard to get here, it is common to listen closely to your body and to wonder what different sensations might mean.

Spotting and bleeding

Spotting is common in early pregnancy. Light bleeding can happen as the embryo settles, after a scan or sometimes without a clear reason. Brown blood often indicates older blood leaving the uterus. Fresh red bleeding, particularly if it becomes heavy or is accompanied by pain, is more concerning. If bleeding changes in colour or volume, or if you are not sure whether to worry, contact your clinic or Early Pregnancy Unit. You do not have to assess this alone.

CASE STUDY: MIA AND JOSH, AND THEIR SCARE DURING THE TWO-WEEK WAIT

Mia had spotting four days before the end of her two-week wait. It began as light brown discharge and then became pink. She described feeling sure her period was coming, and she spent several hours replaying the treatment cycle in her mind, trying to work out what she could have done differently. Josh stayed hopeful, but Mia felt she needed to prepare herself for a negative result.

She tested on the planned day and was surprised to see a faint positive. The spotting continued into early pregnancy, sometimes stopping for a day and then returning. Their clinic arranged a blood test to check hormone levels. Her hCG was rising as expected, but her progesterone was lower than they hoped to see, so the clinic increased her medication.

The spotting eased gradually, although it did not stop completely until around eight weeks. Their first scan showed a pregnancy in the uterus with a visible heartbeat. Mia cried quietly, surprised by her own relief. Josh said it was the first time the pregnancy felt real.

Looking back, Mia described those early weeks as a lesson in uncertainty. She said she learned that spotting can happen even when everything is progressing normally, and that needing medication adjustments does not mean the pregnancy is failing. Their baby was born the following spring.

Pregnancy loss

Sometimes, a pregnancy does not continue. This is called miscarriage/pregnancy loss. It can happen early, or it may be found during a scan without warning. Neither scenario reflects anything you did or did not do. It is something biological that changed. The emotional impact can be profound. Please know that if this becomes part of your story, care and support exist.

Radical honesty: If loss ever becomes part of your story, you may hear phrases like 'At least it was early', 'At least you know you can conceive' or 'It is just one of those things'. People often say these things hoping to comfort you, but they can feel dismissive when you have suffered a loss. Early miscarriage is still a loss. You are allowed to feel what you feel without shrinking it for others.

Ectopic pregnancy

On rare occasions, an embryo implants outside the uterus, most often in a fallopian tube. This is called an ectopic pregnancy. It requires prompt medical attention. Symptoms can include one-sided abdominal pain, shoulder tip pain, dizziness or faintness or bleeding that does not settle. If any of these appear, seek urgent medical help. Early treatment protects your health and future fertility.

> **Radical honesty: Fear in early pregnancy is not a sign of negativity. It is a sign of love and investment. When something matters deeply, the mind looks for what could threaten it. Knowing what to look out for is an act of care, not pessimism.**

If uncertainty or loss becomes part of your journey, you are not expected to navigate it alone.

The emotional landscape

Early pregnancy after fertility treatment can sit in a delicate middle space. You have reached something you hoped for, worked for, maybe longed for. Yet the mind often takes time to believe what the body has already done. You may feel joy, caution, calmness or fear. You may feel several of these in the same day, or you might feel very little at first. All of these responses are within the range of normal.

Many people describe early pregnancy as a period of waiting. Waiting for blood results, waiting for a scan, waiting for the next reassuring sign. When the journey to get here has been long or uncertain, trust often grows in small steps. It is quite normal not to feel confident immediately.

Connection can develop gradually. Some people bond quickly. Others wait for scans, for symptoms or for a sense of safety they cannot quite locate yet. You do not have to love the pregnancy from the first moment. You do not have to speak about the future before you feel ready. You are still allowed to be protective of your hope.

There may also be moments of surprise. Realising you are thinking ahead without noticing. Imagining a milestone you once avoided picturing. Finding yourself placing a hand on your belly without meaning to. These small moments carry meaning too, even if they arrive quietly.

You may find yourself checking for symptoms or looking for signs that they are still there. Symptoms can fluctuate. They can disappear and return. They can stay mild throughout early pregnancy. None of this gives a reliable answer about how things are progressing.

> **Radical honesty: Early pregnancy after treatment is rarely one emotion. It can be relief layered with caution, happiness held**

alongside fear, hope that feels careful. You do not need to resolve these tensions. You only need to keep moving one step at a time.

If you notice that you are comparing yourself with other people's experiences, gently remind yourself that pregnancy stories unfold differently. Some share early. Some wait. Some tell no one for now. You do not have to follow a rule. You are allowed to choose what feels safe for you.

If you find the waiting heavy or if anxiety begins to take up space, it can help to ground yourself in the present rather than fast-forward to outcomes. A short practice might be placing a hand over your chest, taking one slow breath and naming something true for today. You are pregnant. It is early. You are not expected to know more than this right now.

Support

You do not need to move through these weeks bravely or neatly. Early pregnancy can be tender, uncertain or even surreal. Support at this stage is not about fixing anything. It is about having places you can land when you need to.

Support might come from one trusted person. It might come from a partner, a friend you can message at midnight or someone who has been through fertility treatment and understands the language of waiting. It might come from a therapist, or from a quiet moment alone when you let your shoulders drop.

Radical honesty: You can choose how much you share and when you share it. It is about what feels safe for you.

If worry rises, you can ask for more holding. This might look like an extra scan, a brief call with the clinic, a conversation with a counsellor or simply naming out loud that this feels big. You are not expected to feel steady all the time.

Radical honesty: In the first trimester, whatever you need is exactly what you need. If you need more scans, ask for them. If you need time off work, take it. If you need to step back from social media, do so. If you need distraction, connection, privacy or stillness, follow that instinct. The only non-negotiable here is self-kindness.

There is no right way to be pregnant after treatment. There is only your way. One step, one scan, one day at a time is enough.

Final thoughts

Pregnancy after IVF is often described as the moment you finally 'get there', but in reality, it marks the beginning of a new chapter with its own set of emotions and uncertainties. The path to conception through assisted reproduction is rarely straightforward, and reaching a positive test after all of that effort is a significant milestone, but it does not erase the complexity that follows. Transitioning from fertility treatment into routine pregnancy care can feel unfamiliar, sometimes grounding and sometimes unsettling, and it is completely normal to move through this phase with mixed feelings.

Pregnancy after fertility treatment asks something delicate of you. It invites hope while quietly reminding you of everything it took to get here. You may notice that the milestones others seem to move through easily feel different for you. Announcing a pregnancy might take more thought. Buying tiny clothes or allowing yourself to imagine the future may come more slowly, or only after certain points have passed. These experiences are not signs of detachment or doubt. They reflect a journey that has involved risk, effort and waiting.

And yet, success stories unfold every day. Babies are born to people who once sat exactly where you are sitting now. Some of the most meaningful moments in our work have been when people returned months later, baby in arms. We held those babies after holding their parents through stimulation, embryo transfers, disappointment, recovery, patience and trying again. It never stopped being extraordinary.

We cannot promise outcomes; no one can. But we can hold hope with you in a steady, grounded way. Your journey already speaks of resilience. Your body is growing something new. Each week offers fresh evidence, strength and momentum.

Wherever this chapter leads, you deserve to move through it with care and without rushing yourself. You can allow space for gentleness when you need it and permission to pause when things feel heavy. You can decide how much you share, whom you lean on and how you protect yourself as you move forwards. We hope this chapter supports you in doing that, and in whatever comes next for you and that, little by little, this next chapter begins to feel less frightening and more exciting than you ever imagined possible.

Final thoughts and encouragement for those going through treatment

As you close this book, place a hand on your heart for a moment. Notice your breath. Notice the weight of everything you have survived in order to be here, reading these words. You have already shown more resilience than you may ever give yourself credit for.

You do not have to know what comes next. You only have to meet the day you are in.

If you need hope, take a little from us.
If you need rest, take it without apology.
If you need support, reach for it; you deserve it.
If you need belief, borrow ours for now.
You are not alone in this. You never were. You never will be.

Stay positive, and if you cannot, stay patient. Fertility treatment can be a rollercoaster of emotions with its highs and lows.

Seek support. Do not hesitate to lean on your support network, whether it's your partner, family, friends or a support group. Sharing your feelings and experiences can provide immense comfort and strength.

> **Radical honesty: Many people find it surprisingly hard to ask for support during fertility treatment. You may feel like you should stay strong, keep going or manage things quietly on your own. But this journey can feel lighter when shared with people you trust, even in small ways. You do not have to carry every thought or emotion by yourself.**

Educate yourself. Understanding the IVF process, procedures and potential outcomes can alleviate anxiety and help you to make informed decisions. Ask questions, and seek information from your fertility clinic or trusted sources.

Take care of yourself. Self-care is crucial during this time. Focus on maintaining a healthy lifestyle, including a nutritious diet, regular exercise and managing stress through relaxation techniques or hobbies you enjoy.

Embrace emotional support. Consider counselling or therapy to navigate the emotional challenges of IVF. Professional support can provide coping strategies and a safe space to express your feelings.

Celebrate milestones. Acknowledge and celebrate each step of your IVF journey, whether you are starting a new treatment cycle, reaching retrieval or transfer milestones or receiving positive news. Every small victory counts.

You do not have to always be able to do this, but when it is appropriate, remember the hope. Remember that advancements in reproductive technology continue to improve success rates.

Be kind to yourself. IVF can bring forth a range of emotions, from hope and excitement to disappointment and frustration. Be gentle with yourself, and allow yourself to feel whatever emotions come up.

Keep communication open. Maintain open communication with your fertility specialist. They are there to support you and answer your questions.

> **Radical honesty: It is your fertility specialist's job to make sure you feel held and taken care of.**

Believe in your strength. You are stronger and more resilient than you may realise.

A FINAL AFFIRMATION

'Even though I feel anxious/scared/numb/terrified/overwhelmed/stressed/tired/over it/angry/sad/ _______, I am doing the very best I can.'

We know that you are.
Jules and Louise x

APPENDIX 1

List of common fertility-related acronyms and abbreviations

Common terms

AFC: antral follicle count
AI: artificial intelligence
AMH: anti-Müllerian hormone
ART: assisted reproductive technology
ASRM: American Society for Reproductive Medicine
BMI: body mass index
DHEA: dehydroepiandrosterone
DHEAS: dehydroepiandrosterone sulphate
EMMA: endometrial microbiome analysis
ERA: endometrial receptivity array
ESHRE: European Society of Human Reproduction and Embryology
FET: frozen embryo transfer
GABA: gamma-aminobutyric acid
GnRH: gonadotrophin-releasing hormone
HCQ: hydroxychloroquine
HFEA: Human Fertilisation & Embryology Authority
HSG: hysterosalpingography
ICB: Integrated Care Board
ICSI: intracytoplasmic sperm injection
IUI: intrauterine insemination
IVF: in vitro fertilisation
IVIG: intravenous immunoglobulin
LIT: lymphocyte immunisation therapy
MRI: magnetic resonance imaging
NAD: nicotinamide adenine dinucleotide
NK: natural killer
OHSS: ovarian hyperstimulation syndrome
OPK: ovulation predictor kits
PMOS: polyendocrine metabolic ovarian syndrome
PGT: preimplantation genetic testing
PID: pelvic inflammatory disease
PRP: platelet-rich plasma
SHBG: sex hormone binding globulin
STI: sexually transmitted infections
TPO: thyroid peroxidase
TSH: thyroid-stimulating hormone
TTC: trying to conceive
WHO: World Health Organization

Hormones and tests

AMH: anti-Müllerian hormone
E2: oestradiol (a form of oestrogen)
FSH: follicle-stimulating hormone
hCG: human chorionic gonadotrophin
HSG: hysterosalpingography
LH: luteinising hormone
P4: progesterone

Procedures and treatments

ET: embryo transfer
PGT: preimplantation genetic testing
PGT-A: preimplantation genetic screening (previously known as PGS)
PGT-M: preimplantation genetic diagnosis (previously known as PGD)
MESA: microsurgical epididymal sperm aspiration
SA: semen analysis
TESA: testicular sperm aspiration
TESE: testicular sperm extraction

Pregnancy terms

BFN: big fat negative (negative pregnancy test)
BFP: big fat positive (positive pregnancy test)
CD: cycle day
DPO: days past ovulation
DP3DT: days past three-day transfer
DP5DT: days past five-day transfer
EDD: estimated due date
MC: miscarriage
OPK: ovulation predictor kit

Miscellaneous

2WW: two-week wait
AF: Aunt Flo (menstruation)
AI: artificial insemination
AIH: artificial insemination with husband
BBT: basal body temperature
BD: baby dance (intercourse)
CB: cycle buddy
CF: cycle fluid
CM: cervical mucus
DE: donor egg
DOR: diminished ovarian reserve
DPR: days post-retrieval
DPT: days post-transfer
EPT: early pregnancy test
ET: embryo transfer
FP: follicular protocol
FM: fertile mucus
FV: fertile vibes
GC: gestational carrier
HPT: home pregnancy test
IF: infertility
LO: Love Olympics (sex)
LSP: low sperm count
LPD: luteal-phase defect
MF: male factor
O, Ov: ovulation
OD: ovulation dysfunction
OPT: ovulation predictor test
OTC: over the counter
PG: pregnant
PUPO: pregnant until proven otherwise
POAS: pee on a stick
PI: primary infertility
POI: progesterone in oil
RE: reproductive endocrinologist
RPL: recurrent pregnancy loss

APPENDIX 2

Glossary

Acupuncture: A complementary therapy involving the insertion of thin needles into specific points on the body. It is believed to increase blood flow to reproductive organs, regulate hormones and reduce stress during fertility treatments like IVF.

AI (artificial intelligence): Technology applied in IVF to analyse data and predict egg and embryo quality, optimise treatment plans and improve success rates by making IVF more personalised and precise.

Alcohol and drug use: Substances such as alcohol and recreational drugs can negatively affect fertility by disrupting hormonal balance, reducing sperm quality and increasing the risk of pregnancy loss. Moderation or abstinence is advisable during IVF.

Beta hCG (beta human chorionic gonadotrophin): A hormone produced by the developing placenta that is measured to confirm pregnancy and monitor its progression after IVF. Rising levels typically indicate a healthy pregnancy.

Blastocyst: An embryo that has developed for five days after fertilisation, typically at the stage where it is ready for implantation in the uterine lining during IVF.

Case study: A real-life example used to illustrate how a couple or individual navigates fertility treatment or IVF, including challenges faced and solutions found.

CBT (cognitive behavioural therapy): A psychological therapy that focuses on identifying and changing negative thought patterns and behaviours, useful for reducing stress, anxiety and depression during fertility treatments.

Chromosomal abnormalities: Anomalies in the number or structure of chromosomes in embryos, which can lead to genetic disorders or failure of the embryo to implant. Screening for these abnormalities is possible through genetic testing in IVF.

Cryopreservation: The process of freezing eggs, sperm or embryos for future use, preserving reproductive cells for those undergoing medical treatments or delaying family planning.

Cycle monitoring: The regular observation of hormone levels, follicle development and the uterine lining during an IVF cycle. Monitoring helps adjust medication dosages and time-critical procedures like egg retrieval.

Dietary supplements: Vitamins and minerals like folic acid, vitamin D and omega-3 are often recommended to support fertility by improving egg and sperm health, hormonal balance and overall reproductive wellbeing.

Ectopic pregnancy: A serious condition in which a fertilised egg implants outside the uterus, most commonly in the fallopian tube. Symptoms include sharp abdominal pain, vaginal bleeding and dizziness. It requires urgent medical attention.

Egg freezing (oocyte cryopreservation): A procedure that involves freezing and storing eggs for future use, allowing women to preserve their fertility, especially before undergoing medical treatments or when choosing to delay pregnancy.

Embryo grading: A process in IVF where embryos are evaluated based on their appearance, cell division and other factors to assess their potential for successful implantation and development into a pregnancy.

Embryo transfer: The procedure where a fertilised embryo is placed into the uterus for potential implantation and pregnancy during IVF treatment.

Equivocal beta hCG: A beta hCG result that falls in a grey area, often between 5 and 25mIU/ml, where it is unclear if pregnancy is progressing or may result in pregnancy loss.

Fertility preservation for cancer patients: Freezing eggs, sperm or embryos to protect fertility before undergoing treatments like chemotherapy that may harm reproductive tissues.

Fibroids: Non-cancerous growths made of muscle and fibrous tissue that develop in the wall of the uterus. They are common and often cause no symptoms, but depending on their size and location they can sometimes affect the space where an embryo implants and a pregnancy develops.

Folic acid: A B-vitamin that is essential for healthy cell division and is recommended to support fertility and prevent neural tube defects in early pregnancy.

Fragmentation: In embryo development, fragmentation refers to the presence of cellular debris in embryos, which may indicate stress or developmental issues that potentially impact embryo quality.

Genetic screening (preimplantation genetic testing, or PGT): Testing embryos for chromosomal abnormalities or genetic disorders before implantation during IVF, improving success rates and reducing the risk of passing genetic conditions to offspring.

Gluten-free diet: A diet free from wheat, barley and rye, which some people adopt during fertility treatments due to concerns about gluten's impact on inflammation and fertility, though research is still ongoing.

hCG (human chorionic gonadotrophin): A hormone produced during early pregnancy and measured in IVF to confirm pregnancy and monitor its progression.

Hormone monitoring: Regular blood tests to measure levels of hormones like progesterone and oestrogen, which help track the progress of fertility treatments and ensure that the uterus is ready for implantation.

ICSI (intracytoplasmic sperm injection): A laboratory technique used during IVF where a single sperm is injected directly into an egg to help fertilisation occur. It is often used when there are concerns about sperm number, movement or shape.

IUI (intrauterine insemination): A fertility treatment where sperm are directly placed into the uterus during ovulation to increase the chances of fertilisation.

IVF (in vitro fertilisation): A procedure where eggs are fertilised with sperm outside the body, and embryos are transferred to the uterus to achieve pregnancy.

Lifestyle factors: Behaviours that affect fertility, such as diet, alcohol consumption, smoking, exercise and stress management. Maintaining a healthy lifestyle is critical for both partners in the fertility journey.

Mindfulness: A mental practice of being fully present in the moment, often involving techniques like meditation and deep breathing. Often used to reduce stress during fertility treatment.

Minimal stimulation protocols: IVF treatments with milder ovarian stimulation aimed at retrieving fewer eggs with lower hormone dosages, reducing the physical burden on patients.

Mock cycle: A preparatory step in IVF, where some or all treatment steps are simulated to help personalise the actual IVF cycle. This allows doctors to observe how the body responds to medications.

Multiple pregnancies: Pregnancies involving more than one fetus, often resulting from fertility treatments like IVF, which increase the likelihood of twins or triplets.

OHSS (ovarian hyperstimulation syndrome): A condition that can occur during fertility treatments when the ovaries respond excessively to hormonal stimulation, causing symptoms like bloating, nausea and abdominal pain.

Ovarian stimulation: A process in IVF where hormones are used to stimulate the ovaries to produce multiple eggs. This step is crucial for retrieving a sufficient number of mature eggs for fertilisation.

Personalised medicine: Tailoring fertility treatments based on individual patient needs, medical history and genetic profiles to improve IVF outcomes and reduce unnecessary interventions.

Preimplantation genetic testing (PGT): A technique used during IVF to screen embryos for genetic disorders or chromosomal abnormalities before implantation, improving success rates.

Progesterone: A hormone crucial for preparing the uterine lining for embryo implantation and supporting early pregnancy. It is often supplemented during IVF to help maintain pregnancy.

Radical honesty: A recurring term used to highlight candid, sometimes difficult truths about the emotional and physical challenges of IVF and fertility treatments.

Sperm collection: The process of providing a sperm sample, often through masturbation, to be used in IVF or IUI treatments. Samples are tested for motility, count and quality.

Stem cell technology: Research into the potential of using stem cells to create viable eggs and sperm, offering new possibilities for those with fertility issues that currently have no available solutions.

Support system: A network of family, friends, counsellors or support groups that provide emotional and practical help during fertility treatment.

Trigger shot: An injection given during fertility treatments to trigger the final maturation of eggs before they are retrieved for IVF or IUI.

Ultrasound scans: Imaging technology used to monitor egg development, embryo growth and uterine conditions during fertility treatments, ensuring that all stages are progressing as expected.

Wearable technology: Devices such as smartwatches or fitness trackers used to monitor health data. In IVF, these devices can track hormone levels and lifestyle factors, and can provide real-time insights to support personalised treatment.

APPENDIX 3

Resources

For further reading and support, the following resources can be helpful:

- NHS Fertility Treatments: Comprehensive information on available treatments and services.
- Fertility Network UK: Support, information and advice for those experiencing fertility problems.
- RESOLVE: The National Infertility Association: Advocacy and support for those dealing with infertility.

Our favourite Instagram handles

@the_worst_girlgang_ever
@theofficialelizabethking
@sanazghazalmd
@nataliecrawfordmd
@lisa.penny.fertilityism
@eliananutritionuk
@parenthoodinmind
@twolinesfertility
@definingmum
@fertilily_help_hub
@fertility.theribbonbox
@hilariously_infertile
@infertilityfriends
@itmightnotbeheritmightbeyou
@ivf.babymaker
@ivfbabble
@modernfertility
@Myfertility.life
@Plan Your Baby
@pregnantish
@proovtest
@sprinklebabydust
@the.ivf.guide
@the.ivf.warrior

Index